. . . .

"Joe and Sarah have added a comprehensive look and guide to help us understand the importance of lasting love and the power of **Vitamin C**—our crucial life force that is **Connection**. By focusing on the romantic and helping unpack things that interfere with ongoing "love" relationships, *Battles of the Sexes* is a very useful guide to help us stay together and thrive as couples rather than just making it through."

John Ratey, Author of *Go Wild* and *Spark*

"*Battles of the Sexes* takes the latest science of relationships and turns it into cogent advice on how to build happy and healthy long-term relationships. This useful and fun-to-read guide is great for anyone looking for a relationship or who wants to improve their current relationship."

Paul J. Zak, PhD, Author of
The Moral Molecule and *Trust Factor*

"We hear a lot about the 'birds and the bees,' but all too often, the knowledge of most people stops at the plumbing (at best), leaving out the most crucial and sexy part of the human body: between the ears. *Battles of the Sexes* does a wonderful job exploring this crucial part of human nature—our evolutionary inheritance with regard to sexual behavior. Read it and your SEX IQ will soar!"

David P. Barash, Author of *Out of Eden*

"Dr. Joe Malone and Sarah Harris MS, RDN have compiled years of outstanding research to present an engaging text that captures the essence of human relationships and encourages the evolution of companionship through self-actualization. A must-read to improve the interactions with the world around us!"

Amity Parker, RN, Tennessee Oncology

"*Battles of the Sexes* highlights important struggles that should be talked about and understood in a young adult's life. It is truly enlightening and almost like a manual for young men and women to read and understand themselves more. As the world around us changes, so do our battles. It is vital to know how to equip yourself against the negative impacts of the 21st century. This book does just that and more."

Ashley Conway, Vanderbilt University Center for Research on Health Disparities

"Having been coached by Dr. Joe many years ago in my late teens and early 20's to prepare for a Stanford education and four years of collegiate football, I can absolutely attest to his ability to help prepare one's self for the road ahead, especially in those formative years. And this was long before he began his journey of advanced education and research that led to *Battles of the Sexes*!

"This book helps us understand how our biochemistry has such a profound influence on our behavior and relationships, particularly in young adults. In a format that brings a complex subject to enjoyable layman's terms, Dr. Joe explains how our human biological makeup creates sexual conflict and tension in our relationships. Understanding this dynamic between biology and behavior can promote a healthier society for generations to come by reducing destructive behaviors in both men and women. While the emphasis here may be young adults, all ages can benefit and learn from this book. I look forward to applying the knowledge obtained here to my own marriage!

Steve Lemon, Vice President, Trading and Sales, Ross, Sinclaire & Associates

"In today's environment, there might not be a hotter topic then sexual misconduct. *Battles of the Sexes* looks at the sexes in new and resourceful ways, and gives you a behind-the-scenes look at everything that we know, and things we thought we knew, to work as a guide to the background of human sexuality behavior."

Paul Wydra, MS, University Director of Development Initiatives

"Dr. Joe Malone draws some very powerful and fundamental points in *Battles of the Sexes,* insights that we should all take heed of in today's world. As a marriage and family therapist, I know that education is paramount in the quest for more successful sexual and interpersonal relationships. And since we're all biological beings, it would only stand to reason that fighting against our biological urges and predispositions can't bode well for us. *Battles of the Sexes* is a much-needed resource that's missing from the current narrative on human reproductive nature. Touching upon so many topics relevant to society today, such as poor nutrition, overabundance of stress, lack of sleep and our dependence on electronic communication devices, Dr. Joe Malone and Sarah Harris have started a conversation that's not only crucial, but also required, in order for us to understand and repair our relationships with sex and with each other. This book will no doubt help to lead us all in our quest for lower sexual conflict and empowering, long-lasting relationships."

Dr. Isabell Springer, Marriage and Relationship Therapist, Founder of LovEd

"In *Battles of the Sexes*, Malone and Harris have accomplished what few sex educators before them have—namely, they have shown how an understanding of evolutionary principles can improve the sexual and romantic lives of young people. Although one can argue with their conclusions, their effort to take biology seriously as a foundation for all subsequent discussion of sexuality and its pitfalls should be applauded."

Dr. Greg Gorelik

"Finally, a book for college-aged men and women that explains the natural motives that drive relationship behavior differences between men and women that often seem "un-natural" to the opposite sex and at times even us. *Battles of the Sexes* has a laugh out loud effect because of it's true scientific view of the hidden world just beneath the skin of men and women that controls the basics for the survival or our species; the complementary balance between sex-specific behaviors, sex drive, the value of relationships, and holistic health for the present and future generations."

Erin V.L. Smith, PhD Candidate, Founder of Imprinted Legacy

"Almost three decades ago, I met Joe Malone and quickly came to appreciate his work and expertise as a personal trainer. All these years later, I respect and appreciate even more his consistent commitment to improving the health and well-being of individuals, especially young people."

Carol Etherington, Past President Doctors Without Borders, Associate Professor Emerita, Vanderbilt University School of Nursing, Vanderbilt Institute for Global Health

"Battles of the Sexes: Rasing Sexual IQ to Lower Sexual Conflict and Empower Lasting Love provides a unique way to examine relationships and how they relate to overall health. Backed with scientific evidence, it is a great resource for couples of any age to revamp relationships and individual well-being."

Lauren Davis, Operating Room Registered Nurse

"As a former student of Dr. Malone and a single male millennial I can attest that the guidance and knowledge that Dr. Malone presents is both sincere and practical. We all must face ourselves in the pursuit of love and happiness, however armed with the tools here in Battles of the Sexes, we all have a clear advantage in achieving self mastery and romantic success and longevity."

Austin Ellis, Music Artist, NBC's The Voice, Season 6

Battles of the Sexes

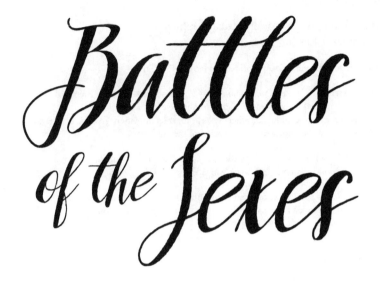

Battles of the Sexes

Raising Sexual IQ to Lower Sexual Conflict
and Empower Lasting Love

DR. JOE MALONE
Sarah Harris, MS, RDN

NEW YORK

LONDON • NASHVILLE • MELBOURNE • VANCOUVER

Battles of the Sexes

Raising Sexual IQ to Lower Sexual Conflict and Empower Lasting Love

Published in New York, New York, by Morgan James Publishing. Morgan James is a trademark of Morgan James, LLC. www.MorganJamesPublishing.com

The Morgan James Speakers Group can bring authors to your live event. For more information or to book an event visit The Morgan James Speakers Group at www.TheMorganJamesSpeakersGroup.com.

ISBN 9781683508779 paperback
ISBN 9781683508786 eBook
Library of Congress Control Number: 2017918494

Cover Design by:
Megan Whitney
megan@creativeninjadesigns.com

Interior Design by:
Chris Treccani
www.3dogcreative.net

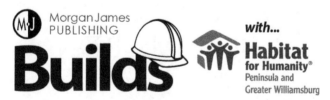

In an effort to support local communities, raise awareness and funds, Morgan James Publishing donates a percentage of all book sales for the life of each book to Habitat for Humanity Peninsula and Greater Williamsburg.

Get involved today! Visit
www.MorganJamesBuilds.com

Table of Contents

. . . .

Foreword

●●●●●●●●

There is no more exciting course to teach than Human Sexuality to college students. One of the things that makes it so exciting is the fantastic pace of change we see every day in our lives involving sex. Upon entering the class, my students walk in with certain beliefs, knowledge, values, and attitudes about sexuality. Many students walk in with personal experiences that often, in their mind, qualify them as experts in the topic. Students also make the assumption when registering for a Human Sexuality class that the entire semester will be all about SEX. Yet the gratification comes when a student asks halfway through the semester, "When we will start discussing sex?" Because it is then that they finally realize there is more to the subject then the actual act.

Most have a misconception about what sexuality is. The word "SEXUALITY" is not just about sex. Certainly, it is a part of it. The first three letters [Sex] demonstrate that. But the ending letters, "UALITY" is about **who we are as sexual beings**. And for people to understand sex, they must first understand themselves. Humans are not born knowing sexuality. Instead, they are conditioned by societal norms, family/friends, ethical, cultural, and psychological factors. And in many instances, those factors can positively AND, more often than not, negatively affect ones view of sex. The first step to diving into this interesting topic is to first understand what sexuality means:

"Sexuality is not only about having sex or taking part in sexual behaviors. Sexuality is about the person you feel you are, your body, how you feel as a boy or girl, man or woman, the way you dress, move and speak, and the way you act and feel about other people. It's not about what you do; it's about who you are and how you live." (SIECUS, 2000).

I often use the analogy that sexuality is like an onion. One must peel back every layer to reach the middle. The layers represent our personal experience, either bad and/or good. Everything that has occurred in life ultimately affects our personal views of sex. And so many times those experiences can leave one's view of sexuality jaded and distorted creating psychological barriers that will affect not only who they believe they are, but their intimate relationships as well. Once a person can understand who they are AND be comfortable with their sexuality, they then understand how it affects their overall well-being. If we start to teach people to value, understand, and love who they are, they in turn allow others to love them. This self-discovery immensely improves the depths of their intimate relationships.

In *Battles of the Sexes*, Dr. Malone's approach is one I greatly admire and is necessary in the field of sexuality. This book utilizes cutting edge, yet understandable science to explain the fundamentals of sexuality starting with the basic biology and differences of both genders. What makes this book different is the detailed, uncomplicated explanation of the female menstrual cycle, female choice, and paternity certainty. It explores the topic of sexual selection, sexual IQ and sexual conflict. And in the typical Coach Malone fashion, he positively infuses sexuality with psychology and guides the reader through conflict resolution.

Dr. Malone is able to integrate his relatable personal experiences with years of research, education, and professional development. In an insightful and compassionate way, the book addresses women's health beginning in the womb and through all stages of sexual development. Chapters devoted to both male and females are informative and instructional, allowing for self-discovery, self-understanding, and understanding of gender differences that will enrich personal relationships.

In sexuality education, KNOWLEDGE IS POWER. What we are finding on the collegiate level is that a large portion of college students come to college with little knowledge of sexuality. The common response when asked what I teach is "you teach sex education to college students? Don't they already know about it?" The answer is no. In my 18 years of teaching Human Sexuality at a large public university, it is my experience that the knowledge they may possess is false and at times just plain absurd.

This generation is falling though the educational cracks. School administrators fail to acknowledge the importance of sexuality education or in most cases do not teach to avoid controversy. Parents rely on schools to teach sex education. Schools expect sex education to be taught at home. All the while teens are being educated by the media. Porn has become a powerful and yet distorted version of sex education for many people. Unfortunately, we live in a society that constantly bombards us with images of sex that have very little to do with healthy sexuality. This is not a time when sexuality should be neglected given that:

- The average male loses his virginity at age 16 and females at 17 years of age
- 1 in 4 has a sexually transmitted infection.

- 1 in 2 sexually active people will contract a sexually transmitted disease by twenty-five years of age.
- People spent 4.3 billion hours on Pornhub last year, which means 21.2 BILLION visitors watched 87.8 billion videos (Fightthenewdrug.org, 2016)

Dr. Malone and Sarah Harris MS, RDN explain all the related issues while also including areas of sexuality not normally addressed such as "Food Traps" and reproductive nutritional needs for both genders. Large amounts of research are devoted to the psychology of eating and how people medicate with food, however little research has been conducted examining why people often replace sex with food.

Battles of the Sexes spoke to me on many levels. I found myself making notes on the manuscript to include in my future lectures. I was mesmerized by new concepts as well as having the experience of being reaffirmed and validated regarding the material I currently teach to my college students. This book is an interesting read, but more importantly it is USEFUL, especially for college undergraduates.

It was my honor to be asked to write the foreword for Joe's book. After 13 years of friendship both professionally and personally, I admire his passion for teaching and health. His gifted spirit leaves the learner fulfilled and enlightened. The depth of his knowledge for all things health is both impressive and valuable. It is my hope that readers will grasp on to his advice and utilize the tools provided in *Battles of the Sexes* that will empower loving, healthy, and lasting intimate relationships for a lifetime.

Shannon Finch Josey, M.S., CHES

Lecturer of Teaching Human Sexuality, MTSU
Health and Human Performance Department
"Behavior Change Workbook" and *MTSU Health and Wellness Lab Manual* Brentwood, TN

Acknowledgements

• • • • • • • • • • • • • • • •

We would like to acknowledge first and foremost our extraordinarily talented editor Aubrey Kosa without whose outstanding efforts, this book would not have been possible. Our acquistions editor Terry Whalin also provided key support and encouragement at the beginning of this project. We also appreciate all of the wisdom and insights shared with us by our Morgan James Publishing leadership team of David Hancock, Jim Howard, Bethany Marshall and Niara Baskerfield. Your experience in the world of publishing has proven invaluable.

We also want to express our heartfelt thanks to Shannon Finch Josey for writing the foreword for *Battles of the Sexes*. Shannon has done a magnificent job at MTSU of educating many thousands of college students on the "birds and the bees". Shannon is known and greatly admired for her fearless, engaging, and insightful ways of making the mysteries of human sexuality fully understandable to her students year after year. She strongly conveys news they can use!

Joe would like to thank all of his students from whom he has always learned more than he was able to teach. He especially wants to thank those that he quoted in *Battles of the Sexes*.

Joe would like to express to Sarah that over a decade ago when she offered to become "my right-hand man" I could not have envisioned how really superb and effective our partnership would become. There have been so many important health promotions we have done over the years and now with the publication of this book we have reached a whole new level in trying to make a positive difference in people's lives. I am humbled and grateful for your unselfish willingness to volunteer all of your tremendous intelligence and talents to everything we have done. I am forever in your debt!

Sarah would like to show appreciation to Joe for his genuine, authentic desire to better the lives of others without fanfare or wish for accolades. She has, to date, not met a more passionate human being that cared so deeply about the whole-body health of his students and those he coaches. And to every teacher and coach in her life and beyond that have taught the art of thinking outside of the box and marching to the beat of a new drum.

Urban Dictionary Definitions

● ● ● ● ● ● ● ● ● ● ● ● ● ● ● ● ● ● ● ●

Sexual Empathy

The ability to understand and respect the perspective of the opposite sex.

Romance

True romance is doing something special or unexpected for someone you love, even though you don't have to. Romance isn't a greeting card, it isn't Valentine's Day, it isn't a box of chocolates, and it certainly isn't a dozen roses (unless you like that sort of thing). Real romance is not what modern society has been taught to think it is. Real romance isn't manufactured. It is completely individual. Romance is for showing the person you love that you're thinking about them. It shouldn't feel forced. There are no limits to romance; it can be shown by a handwritten note, by going for a walk, or even by making someone a sandwich. Romance is something simple and sweet that reminds your partner why they fell in love with you in the first place.

Introduction

• • • • • • • • •

"The fault, dear Brutus, is not in our stars,
but in ourselves"
SHAKESPEARE FROM *JULIUS CAESAR*

"Know thyself"
SOCRATES

Where the Passion Began

With regard to Socrates' famous quote, I, Joe Malone, came to know myself by trial and a boatload of error. As a young adult, I experienced a tumultuous time during the early 1990s. When it was all said and done, I was diagnosed with Obsessive Compulsive Disorder (OCD).

I was first treated through many different versions of Freudian talk therapy, which did not change the OCD symptoms at all.

> **Freudian Theory:** The first psychoanalytic theory developed by Sigmund Freud in the late nineteenth century that emphasized the importance of the unconscious mind and rested on

> the assumption that people are driven fundamentally by
> unconscious, animalistic, instinctual urges, particularly lust (eros)
> and aggression (thanatos), and are influenced by childhood
> events, particularly traumatic ones.

Being continually asked if I had suffered abuse or other negative influences as a child only created frustration, and eventually desperation and depression, as I tried psychologist after psychologist who continued using talk therapies to no avail. The low point was when one psychologist asked me why I *wanted* to have OCD.

(Trust me, anybody who has OCD will tell you that nobody would ever volunteer to have it. It is a torturous condition to endure!)

It was then that I started seeing a psychiatrist (who I learned is a medical doctor with the ability to prescribe medication). She told me that she had a medication she believed would address my symptoms. She began treating me with antidepressant medications.

After several weeks, she proved to be correct.

It wasn't until much later that I learned I was one of the approximately 50 percent of OCD sufferers that also has bipolar disorder. The high daily dosages of antidepressants took me out of the dungeon of depression to the mile-high experience of mania. That mania led to unintentional damage to my life and those around me. I learned painfully and personally in no uncertain terms about the biological chemical reality at the root of the human condition that influences our behavior.

On one hand, I finally got some relief. I learned that what I was suffering from was a biologically-based chemical imbalance in my brain that had *not* come from abusive socialization when I was a child, but from a brain chemistry predisposition I had inherited from my ancestors.

Imagine that.

The bad news was that besides triggering the manic symptoms previously mentioned, the relief from the antidepressants lasted only a few months and I found I had to keep trying new medications as my brain habituated to each one. Eventually, I discovered that a combination of medication plus a new kind of talk therapy called Cognitive Behavioral Therapy are what would finally help bring a level of control to my OCD/bipolar brain condition. Looking back on it, I clearly recognize that the key to gaining control was learning how my own brain and those of others worked on a biochemical basis.

That was the point in my life when I realized that I desperately needed what we would eventually call Sex IQ. This is when the initial seeds were planted and the journey through a world of human biochemical research and related self-discovery began.

Going into the 2000s, as I continued acquiring more and more biochemical knowledge, I was able to holistically manage my own life to the point where I could live successfully with OCD and bipolar disorder. I was able to taper off all medication, which my doctors told me would never be possible.

The key insight I took away from my experience with the treatment of OCD and bipolar disorder is that human behavior is a matter of both nature and nurture. Through the Freudian era, which took up most of the twentieth century, human behavior was thought to be mostly a matter of nurture. It became clear to me that we needed to make good use of knowledge from both the sciences of nature *and* nurture to have the maximum beneficial effect on human behavior. I landed in the midst of the mental health change brought about by the natural scientific breakthroughs in the area of brain function that characterized the 1990s. These fortuitous circumstances happened as a result of changing governmental policy that recognized the importance of understanding the brain on a biological level. The 1990s are still known as the "decade of the brain" because government funding caused an explosion of new knowledge on brain structure and biochemistry. From a highly personally informed and motivated perspective, I began studying the brain and have yet to stop.

As a result of this study, I started understanding life and how my own brain and those of others worked on a biochemical level. Words like dopamine, serotonin, noradrenaline, opioids, and oxytocin came to hold deep meaning for me. This knowledge was not only gained through books and research, but through the personal experiences brought about by the prescribed psychotropic medication I was on to combat OCD and bipolar. I learned experientially and in real time the effects of lowered or raised serotonin, dopamine, etc. Those experiences have led me to deeper insights in almost every area of life, including romance and sex.

Let's Talk About Sex—We Are Not the Same

One of the areas I could not ignore in my research was the distinctly unique biochemistries of the sexes. Just like the 1990s' brain biochemistry research, sex differences research is based on "hard" or natural science. Natural selection is the net that snares all of the dissimilar findings of the biological life sciences and brings them together as a coherent whole.

"Natural Selection: The process whereby organisms better adapted to their environment tend to survive and produce more offspring. The theory of its action was first fully expounded by Charles Darwin and is now believed to be the main process that brings about evolution." ~ Oxford Dictionary

One hallmark portion of natural selection is sexual selection, which is the framework for understanding human sex differences.

I was fascinated to see supporting research with non-human species. The pattern was clear: males and females are different on a biochemical basis throughout animal species. For humans, that pattern is especially true during young adulthood (ages 18-39). Clinical psychologist and researcher Dr. Irina Trofimova has established recently that differences between men and women peak at ages 20-23 and decline gradually as they age[1]. There is a profound variance hormonally at that age between most males and females. This is a major cause of the significant behavioral variances observed during this life stage.

In *Battles of the Sexes*, we make the case that it is important to recognize that young men and women are experiencing life differently during this developmental period, and should be given tailored and customized coaching on how to successfully navigate it. There are some people who think that most differences between human males and females are created by societal pressures. We respect this insight and agree that a certain portion can be explained by plasticity of the brain and societal norms; however, after personal life experience and decades of research, it cannot be ignored that a significant proportion of our behavior as humans is reflective of our unique biology. Each of us is a walking biochemical reaction that is constantly responding to others and our environment. We get to where we are at any particular moment in our lives from a combination of biological genetic inheritance, gender, and sociological influence. To discount or dismiss the biological element would be a profound mistake, and one especially dangerous for females. Allow me to explain.

The Biology of the feMALE

The reason that ignoring the biological influence in a woman's life is more dangerous than ignoring it in a man's life is that research has been done primarily on males and then extrapolated to females.

Why would they do that?

Up until the 1990s, females were thought to be difficult and problematic to work with because of hormonal variations. They were construed by researchers as "smaller men," identical except for genitalia and those pesky hormones that were hard to create a control for in experimental design.

An example of research that proved this physically identical approach dead wrong was the discovery that dosages of Ambien need to be significantly smaller for women than they do for men to avoid the lingering effect and the resulting hazards, including unsafe driving conditions. The female body metabolizes Ambien much more slowly than the male body does. The Society for Women's Health Research has been working to point out the gravity of this insight, especially to women, with the hope that they will see the importance to their well-being. They have been advocating for this since the 1990s and are finally being heard and responded to by the medical community and society. This is one of many testaments to the biological uniqueness of the sexes.

Sex differences are real and important and can contribute to knowing ourselves in constructive and preventive ways. Dr. David Geary, one of the world's foremost researchers on sex differences, put it best:

"I ask those readers who remain unconvinced to reflect on the theory of evolution of which sexual selection is one set of pressures. Evolution is not just another psychological, sociological, or anthropological theory; it has proven to be the unifying meta-theory for all of the life and biological sciences. Eventually, all psychological, sociological, and anthropological models will need to be reconciled with the principles of natural selection and sexual selection. One can choose to be part of this discovery process, or one can let these forthcoming scientific advances pass one by."[2]

Society Plays its Part

As someone who has always highly respected the work of social scientists to the point of becoming one myself, I do not take lightly the ability of social groups to influence our behavior. If I did not believe that people could be changed through the influence of others, the college classes I have taught over the years would be designed very differently. Even so, I have come to realize through both empirical evidence and personal experience that the biochemistry and physiology of our ancestors may also have a profound influence on the behavioral inclinations of the sexes. Understanding ourselves and those around us through knowledge of this phenomenon, along with understanding the social influences, is essential.

Shaping the Future

Why is this so important to grasp, especially for young adults?

It is as a young adult that men and women begin sliding into the bodies that can either make them sick and depressed middle-agers or vibrant and joyful old souls. It is as a young adult that humans begin shaping their long-term future. Robin Marantz Henig and her daughter Samantha Henig describe it in their book *Twentysomething*:

"In 2000, when the Add Health (Adolescent to Adult Health) investigators did a new round of interviews, they found that study subjects who were now young adults aged 18-26, had slipped on 16 of the 20 standard indicators of healthy living. They had started smoking, stopped exercising, stopped eating breakfast, started eating junk food and getting fat, stopped going to the dentist and stopped getting annual check-ups. Compared to their behavior as adolescents, the twenty-something participants in the Add Health study engaged in more binge drinking, marijuana use and hard drug use and had higher rates of sexually transmitted diseases."[3]

It is clear that the formative years after leaving the childhood home are a time when much good can be done through preventive strategies. These strategies can be especially effective when informed by biological insight and clothed in psychosocial wellness approaches.

Another reason young adulthood is such an opportune time to intervene in the typical twenty-first century health deterioration process is brain maturation. Dr. Meg Jay, in her book *The Defining Decade,* points out that through recent science, we now know that there are two growth spurts in the development of the brain. The first takes place in the initial eighteen months of life with the brain creating many more neurons than it can use.

Neurons: Cells that transmit nerve signals.

These are employed for learning skills like crawling, walking, speaking, and eating. Those that aren't used to learn are pruned. The second growth spurt occurs from adolescence through at least the mid-20s. Most of these neurons develop in the frontal lobe, which is the seat of judgement, self-control, and intentionality. In the same way as before, the ones that are used to develop behaviors (good or bad) are kept, while those that are leftover are pruned.[4] This makes young adulthood in particular a crucial time to intervene with preventive strategies that lead young men and women onto a healthy and successful path. Because this is the final development stage of the hardwiring of the brain, these habits will have a tendency to become permanent—for better or worse.

From Bad Habits to Heart Attacks

There is a combination of events and experiences that bring us to where we are in life. In the late 1990s, my experiences had shaped me into a disillusioned fitness professional. It was during this same decade that health problems caused by poor lifestyle choices had increased dramatically in Western societies, and it hit me personally when a client of mine died of a heart attack at age 60 while on vacation in Florida. During his forty-year business career, he had created a corporation and amassed a fortune. Unfortunately, he had been so physically inactive that he had no body or health left with which to enjoy it.

In a related incident, I found out that a dear friend of mine had experienced his first heart attack at 48 years old. He too was a victim of the wealthy businessman's excessive traveling lifestyle. I found myself one unforgettable day eight years later giving him chest compressions as he struggled to live after suffering *another* heart attack. It wasn't like the movies or TV. He was turning colors no human should be, green, purple, etc., and trying hard to breathe to stay alive. After twenty-five of the longest minutes of my life, the EMTs arrived and took over.

Unfortunately, he didn't make it.

I came away from that experience traumatized, and as I said, disillusioned and considering quitting the fitness industry. We were being overwhelmed at that time by the sheer number of people needing our help, but could only work with one at a time. It was a feeble and discouraging way to address a tsunami of bad health and although I was tempted to quit, I determined to continue fighting back for the sake of others' health, and, along the way, discovered the massive potential for reaching young adults in preventive ways to avoid them becoming suffering, future-chronic-disease candidates.

Optimal Health Starts in the Womb

I began teaching at a local university in the early 2000s and found that the energy and enthusiasm of the college students matched my own. It was around this same time that I began to discover the emerging science of fetal programming.

> Fetal programming scientifically explains how conditions inside the mother's womb during pregnancy through epigenetic processes can influence the health of the fetus and the future adult throughout their lives. Those conditions can strongly influence a fetus's chances of developing heart disease, diabetes, stroke, autoimmune disorders, and even cancer. Or, looked at from the positive perspective, it can help prevent all of them.

> **Epigenetics:** The study of changes in organisms caused by modification of gene expression, rather than alteration of the genetic code itself.

The state of young women's health leading up to pregnancy is a strong influencing factor on the future health of a baby. The baby is created, quite literally, from the mother's muscle, bone, and fat.[5] I realized this meant that focusing on health promotion, particularly for young women, could finally produce a formidable weapon in the war against the effects of our unhealthy, twenty-first century environment. With each young woman prospectively having an average of two children, this was finally a way to fight back exponentially against the tide of bad health that the 1980s and 90s had launched. When I was working with one young woman, I was essentially working with three people, which included her probable two future babies. I knew that research also showed that she would be a greater influence on her husband than vice versa and would set the health culture of their future home. This raised the number of benefited individuals to four.

This revelation led me on a course of finding innovative ways to work with the college women demographic. In fact, some colleagues and I eventually designed and implemented a new college women's wellness course that became the subject of my doctoral dissertation research. It was about this time in 2007 that I crossed paths with a remarkable and brilliant young woman: Sarah Harris. When I shared my thoughts and vision with her, she said, "If you ever need a right-hand man, let me know."

That was the beginning of a long and fruitful partnership that started with her as a student in my class and proceeded through many health promotions for college women and continued all the way to the present, where she is now a Registered Dietitian with a Master of Science degree in Clinical Nutrition.

At this point, I will let her speak for herself.

A Word from Sarah

As a student studying Nutrition and Food Science and minoring in Exercise Physiology, I took class after class on nutrition and exercise. Joe Malone's Personal Conditioning class was unlike any other course I took as an undergraduate. I could tell something was different immediately. The science he shared with his students about young men and women's health challenges and the relationship between women's health and reproduction (among so many other topics) were unheard of in my traditional classes and it hit me particularly hard. I was that person he was teaching about, and being a member of a sorority at the time, I had a front row seat viewing the poor health decisions young women (including myself) were making on a daily basis: excessive drinking, pizza at every event, fast food and soda galore from rushing around from event to meeting to class, poor campus food choices, substance and supplement abuses, eating disorders. This is what compelled me to reach out to Coach Joe in the first place nine years ago. He was up to something important and I wanted to be a part of the preventive effort alongside him. He genuinely cares for every person's life that he affects and has such incredible intentionality in his coaching efforts. In Battles of the Sexes, as a now married 28-year-old with two young children, it will be my role to chime in and further qualify Malone's science with real-life situations and provide additional expert insight in regard to practical nutrition advice for young adults.

Reproductive Battles of the Sexes

Through the years of developing a college women's wellness program, part of which entailed teaching them the workings and differences of the biochemistry and structure of young men's brains, I had another realization. With mate selection being one of the brain's highest priorities during young adulthood and looking at the way our society has developed in the twenty-first century,[157] the greatest danger to a young man's well-being revolves around their reproductive capability and functions. I had discovered earlier that young women's greatest health threat is also strongly related to their reproductive capability and functions.

The physiological mechanisms that had worked well for our ancestors could be disastrous for present-day young adults if they did what felt good through nature's call. These gender-distinct young adult dilemmas are what we are naming the "Battles of the Sexes."

You are about to get insights into these largely little-known and underappreciated battles and their challenges and opportunities in Part I of *Battles of the Sexes*.

In Part II, we will take a close look at human sexual chemistry and its ramifications.

Part III will examine the more well-known and traditional battle *between* the sexes. This sexual conflict, as we will refer to it, will be explored, along with how all of this battle between the sexes relates to the health and wellbeing of young adults.

Finally, in Part IV, we will take a focused look at the college situation as it eventually leads to the time when most young adults get married (on average, in a young adult's late 20s). I will also use research I have personally conducted to further illuminate insights in the book. There is a progressive nature to the chapters, but also care has been taken to make the information in most chapters stand independently on its own in case you're just interested in reading about a particular topic.

Enhanced knowledge of these battles between our human sexual nature and our twenty-first century culture will raise your sex IQ and lower sexual conflict in your life and those of others.

With all due respect to people of other sexual orientations, it should be noted that we will focus in this book on heterosexuality. There are several reasons for this. One is that we have very little research background and no personal experience in other areas of human sexuality and would feel better having others do the writing in those areas. Also, this book is about the development of humans through natural and sexual selection. These forces, and especially sexual selection, have largely acted on child-producing unions to form the genes that we have today. Therefore, relationships that have the organic physical capability of producing biological offspring are what we are focusing on. That is the heart of the knowledge we share here.

As will be outlined in more detail later, this book was written in consultation with the Sexual Assault Center of Nashville. One of our primary goals is to decrease the amount of sexual violence throughout Western societies. A great deal of sexual violence is created out of sexual conflict between the sexes, which will also be explained in detail later. For that matter, as we will see, much of violence in general in our Western societies is also related. We aim to bring about greater understanding, peace, and harmony between the sexes. For all of these reasons, we focus on heterosexuality in this book.

As a result, if you are a young, heterosexual adult (18-39), you will know yourself better from the genetic level up after reading *Battles of the Sexes*. If you are not, you will still be better able to help and advise those who are, especially those you love.

—————————— A SARAH SUMMARY: ——————————

- We are products of fetal programming, natural and sexual selection, and the experiences and environmental influences of our growth periods.
- Males and females are different on a biochemical basis throughout animal species; to ignore this fact can prove detrimental to society.
- The physiological reproductive mechanisms that worked for our ancestors can be disastrous for twenty-first century young adults who follow their natural urges.

PART I

· · · · ·

The Battles Against
the Mismatch

Chapter 1

· · · · · · · ·

Major Battles of the Sexes: Junk Food & Junk Sex

"The chief purpose of education is to teach young people
the right things to find pleasure in."
PLATO

Shared Battles of the Sexes

Discovery of the Common Battles

From the dawn of human history, we men and women have depended on each other for our mutual success and, yes, even our mutual survival. Quite literally we would not still be here as a species if this was not so. There has had to be a certain amount of sexual empathy, sexual respect, and sexual synergy for a long time for us to be where we are today.

Yet, over the last several decades it seems there has been a growing inability in some quarters of Western society to see the strengths and talents in the other sex. Some women would agree with the phrase "women are from Earth and men are from somewhere close to Uranus." To some degree they have a point. I know as a man there are many things I have said and done that I would like to take back. On the other hand, as is the case for all humans, women aren't perfect either (except for my wife). Some men think that women are manipulative and less than honest in their relationships. I am sure there are also women out there who would like to take back some of the things they have said or done.

Whatever happened to the sentiment of 'can't we all just get along?'

Could much of this negativity come from a colossal nature-nurture-based misunderstanding between the sexes that we may now have the scientific knowledge to clear up? Specifically, could both sexes be victims of, and be struggling and battling with, ancient drives and inclinations that no longer match modern culture and that can cause damage to the other sex? Could education about the human sexual nature each of us has inherited be helpful in this regrettable situation?

We strongly believe this to be the case.

A major hope of *Battles of the Sexes* is to be a uniting and reconciling force between women and men. We believe that women and men are all in this thing called life *together* in the twenty-first century and always have been in it together. As a result, we hope to educate adults (especially young adults) on healthy relationships and in so doing raise their sexual empathy, sexual respect, and ultimately their sexual synergy in everyday friendly relationships with members of the opposite sex, and eventually within the context of romantic love relationships.

I didn't start out aiming to be an educator, and especially not one focused on such crucial matters for humankind and the human heart. My childhood career goal was to become a lawyer. After marrying early, I quickly discovered that law school and matrimony did not necessarily work well together in my life. My fallback plan was obtaining a fifth-year teaching certification.

At first, I spent my days trying to survive teaching in order to get to the best part of my day, which was coaching after-school athletics. I didn't consider myself to be a very good teacher at the time, but as the months went on I began to finally realize the potential for good that could be accomplished with these students in the seven and a half hours I had them in class each day. One of my colleagues observed the enthusiasm and passion with which I coached athletics, and suggested I try some of that in the classroom. I did, and it made a world of difference. From then on, I made coaching in the classroom my signature method. That transformation is important because along the way, I realized the importance of Plato's assertion as quoted at the beginning of this chapter and shaped my coaching style of teaching in a way that strived to teach young people the right things to find pleasure in. The well-being of my students became my passion and remains so to this day.

Discovering how to shape young people's behaviors to benefit their health has become immensely more important as society has morphed into the twenty-first century. Owing to the way that the twenty-first century environment causes both genders to go against their genetic code and biological design, there are some battles that young women and young men may have in common. In their book, *Go Wild*, John Ratey and Richard Manning state that rather than diseases of civilization, a more apt term would be injuries of civilization.[6] They list the results from a study by the Bill and Melinda Gates Foundation showing the top twelve risk factors for disease from 187 countries around the world in 1990-2010. They are listed in order:

1. High blood pressure

2. Smoking
3. Alcohol
4. Household air pollution
5. Low fruit consumption
6. Obesity
7. High blood sugar
8. Low body weight
9. Air pollution
10. Inactivity
11. High salt intake
12. Low nut and seed consumption[7]

Really, most of what we consider diseases of civilization should more properly be called the afflictions of civilization. These risk factors come from forcing humans into environmental circumstances that our genetic design was not meant to accommodate. These physical effects are equal opportunity destroyers in that they are distributed and reacted to detrimentally by most people, male and female, across our society.

A Word from Sarah: Afflictions of Civilization

It is fascinating to me that over 65 percent of the most common risk factors for diseases of civilization are directly related to the foods and beverages we consume. We are not doing nearly enough as a nation to alter our environment in a positive way to combat the increasing threat it is placing on ourselves and the generations to come. As a clinician, it kills me a little bit inside every time I hear the phrase, "I'm going to die somehow, I might as well die happy enjoying the foods that I love rather than miserable eating the healthy crap." I have heard different variations of this statement far too many times, especially during my time in long-term care. I'm not sure that people quite realize how much they are cutting their life short by making the food choices that they do every day. Not to mention, quality of life is so greatly decreased when you are so big you are unable to take care of your own basic needs.

When kids are brought up in homes that share this mentality, they are at high risk of adopting it, and the cycle of ill health continues. One person's negative attitude about healthy living can effectively cut the lives of future generations short as well. Nobody wants to cut the lives of their children and grandchildren short, but that is essentially what is done when respected adults in the family adopt the mindset that unhealthy foods do no harm. I'm reminded of Alana Thompson from "Here Comes Honey Boo" on TLC from 2014, who was raised in a family with a similar unhealthy attitude towards food. What the attitude creates is a family destined for a host of chronic diseases. The stage in our country is set for one of the most abominable cases of self-destruction the human race has seen to date.

Obesity Observations

Ratey and Manning point out that airports are one of the many venues where these afflictions of civilization are easily observed. The first obvious sign is the level of people struggling with obesity, but they ask us to go deeper and take a look at the fitness and well-being of the non-obese as well.

Do they look content and happy? Do they have sallow and sagging skin and downcast eyes?

They ask us to then think back to the same airport scene twenty years ago. Do the pictures look the same?

Most of us would have to say no; they are markedly different.

They go on to point out an even more insightful irony. They remind us that airports are where we hear incessantly the warnings of the threat of a terrorist attack and the need for constant vigilance in that direction and point out very cogently that these imagined possible damages look tame in comparison to the very real damage to the people we see struggling through the airport. They ask, "Who did this to us? Can a greater threat be imagined to our future well-being as a species than the condition of our people? Can an act of terrorism be imagined that would be more terrible to more people than the injuries we have inflicted on ourselves?"[8]

And, come to find out, the most injurious time in our lives as far as obesity is concerned is during young adulthood.

Statistics from the Behavioral Risk Factor Surveillance Survey show that the largest increases in obesity happen in young adults between the ages of 18-29.[9] Many of these young people are college students at the time. I have seen this semester after semester in my classes, and more so in the last few years. I have especially seen it in the young women that I have worked with, and it is becoming increasingly apparent that at younger ages, this problem is becoming overwhelming to many of them.

Relationship Observations

Another battle that both sexes share due to the twenty-first century environment that might not be quite so obvious, but is just as important, is the transformation to the digital society. A great deal of discretionary time is now used by young adults to stay in touch with their online social circle. Around 4,000 texts per month was the average for most 18-24-year-olds in 2012. This comes out to six or seven texts every waking hour. Long gone are the days when a person's first instinct to contact a friend involved picking up a phone and calling or meeting in person for coffee or traveling to each other's homes to visit. Around two-thirds of US millennials text their friends three times as often as they e-mail, call, or see them in person.[10] This means that young adults are most often having only brief contact with peers that involves no eye contact, no tone of voice, and very little emotion expressed (except as emoticons). Instead of the rich conversation of the past, these texts are made up of a solitary thought—one at a time.

Susan Pinker, in *The Village Effect,* speaks to this area of social and emotional life and its importance—the connections all of us have with the people in our lives. She says that our recent understanding of what is important to promote our health and happiness has been focused on the tangible: food, exercise, drugs, career, and success. We have found out scientifically that tobacco, sugar, salt, trans fat, and obesity shorten our lives, while physical activity, the right diet, and medicine prolong it. Very recently, we have discovered that our relationships, the people we know and care for, are just as important to our well-being. But the type of social contact needed to have this beneficial effect is face-to-face contact.[11]

From life's beginning and at every stage of development, close contact with people affects the way we think, the people we decide to trust, and our monetary investments. These social ties influence our sense of life satisfaction, our brain power, and our resistance to infections and chronic diseases. As new science on diet, exercise, and different types of drugs have created life-changing breakthroughs in recent decades, even newer evidence shows that positive social bonds are just as transformative.[12]

Technological Isolation

It is clear that face-to-face social contact is diminishing in our society. This is especially true for our young adults. Some of them are digital natives and it is hard for them to envision their life without their devices. When I first started teaching college, it was common to walk across campus and make eye contact with passers-by and often say "hello." That scenario is now almost unheard of, with most staring down at their phones while walking with earbuds in. Young adults are becoming more and more isolated from face-to-face social contact. In class, I make a strong point of starting each day with what I call team builders, or relational warmups. Every class session, students (we call them "team members") have to get physically warmed up while interacting in friendly ways with other classmates. I see a major change in their ability to pull this off by the end of each semester. They have learned how to create real social bonds over the course of just thirteen weeks.

I have seen that this "teamness" or sense of "us" has a beneficial effect throughout the class and throughout their lives. Whenever they communicate with me (via email, calling, texting, etc.), they refer to their team name and often they use the Positive Identification each one gives themselves to begin class (a positive adjective that starts with the same first letter of their first name, for instance Cool Callie, Jammin' Jasmine, etc.). This is a big change for them from their typical college class experience as I believe in many classes they never even learn their professor's name, let alone their classmates'.

By the way, Sarah's Positive Identification was "Spicy Sarah"!

A Word from Sarah: One Millennial's View on Isolation

Spicy Sarah here! I remember being a bit uncomfortable at first in Coach's personal conditioning class. There was a lot of hand shaking, direct eye contact, and the entrance of smiling strangers into my personal bubble. But it didn't take much time for the discomfort of it all to wear off and turn into excitement and positive energy. This discomfort was probably due to the fact that my contact with most people was through texting, email, or instant messaging, almost always with people I already knew and was comfortable with. With a digital form of communication, you have time to think before you say something. You can conjure up the perfect response to anything with enough time, and you always appear witty, funny, and friendly.

When you're staring at a stranger face-to-face and are forced to interact on a personal level, it forces you to be on your toes. You have to think faster to communicate. This takes far more mental energy than digitally communicating. Texting is an easy "out" to the mental energy you would otherwise have to expend talking to someone directly, be it by phone or in person. If you're communicating exclusively via digital means, you quickly begin to lose the skill required to actually have those real-time conversations.

Speaking solely from personal experience, this decrease in communication skill leads to social anxiety, which leads to further isolation, which eventually breeds depression and the host of ailments that come with depression.

If you take anything from this, please understand that forcing yourself into social situations that take you out of your comfort zone and communicating with strangers or people that are different from you is a beneficial activity and should be practiced on a regular basis.

Dealt a Bad Economic Hand

Andy Preisler, millennial blogger, writes about a final area that both young adult women and men are challenged with in the twenty-first century. He says, "Baby Boomers are upset with today's young adults. They are seen by them as lazy, lacking a strong work ethic, and not saving money. They are not getting married, having children, or buying homes. On top of all of that, many are perceived as being narcissistic. Gen X-ers have noted as well that millennials have not wanted to play by the rules of the traditional levels of management in corporate America."[13]

He counters the Baby Boomer's view by proposing that the real victims in this situation are the millennials themselves.

Despite being the most highly educated American generation (27 percent have at least Bachelor's degrees), their median annual earnings are $2,000 less on average than their similarly credentialed peers back in 1980. Young adults have less net worth than prior generations at the same age. They are being forced to access their savings for crisis management. They are not investing in 401k plans or independent investments because they were traumatized by the crash of 2008. Many young adults have exorbitant student loan debt. The average is $35,000. Paying back at the minimum rate will keep them in debt for many, many years.[14]

The economy has not picked up to the level it was pre-2008 and there is a higher rate of unemployment and underemployment. With stagnant wages and student loan debt, it would be difficult for millennials to ever save for their retirements. They are starting at lower salaries and may not ever make up the difference over the course of their careers. They will also inherit an ever-increasing level of federal debt and may not ever get social security or Medicare when they do reach retirement. Around 50 percent believe that social security and Medicare will be gone by the time they get there[15]—what hope do they have?

In This Together

The stats above are some of the practical and day-to-day challenges both sexes face in this twenty-first century environment.

They are battles of the sexes that both genders face together. Sarah and I believe that much can be done to help young adults overcome these challenges and we hope to be a part of the solution.

We are now going to shift attention to the gender-specific battles that each sex faces as a result of the way Western society has developed in the twenty-first century. These are the challenges that each gender is most vulnerable to because they are a young man or young woman and have the hormonal and brain structure inherited from generations past.

These are the classic battles of the sexes.

Gender-Specific Battles of the Sexes

Hormones 'R Us

As Dr. Irina Trofimova and other researchers have shown, men and women's hormonal profiles are profoundly different during their young adult years (ages 18-39).[16] These differences in hormones produce obvious behavioral differences. It is true that there are some additional influences from society that reinforce these differences through sex role expectations, but as previously stated, the lion's share of deviations seems to emanate from nature rather than nurture.

These variances center on increasing the chances of young men and young women's reproductive success. In ancestral times, the programmed instinctual behavior these innate tendencies compel proved beneficial to each gender for being successful at passing on its genes to the next generation. In the twenty-first century, these same innate drives can lead to young adults destroying their own well-being and lives.

It can be very difficult during youthful years to do the right thing when instincts are pushing in the opposite direction. In many cases, young women and young men may find themselves forming negative habits in the very areas of their lives that they most want to form good ones. These battles of the sexes especially take shape for young men in the area of relationships and young women in the areas of fitness and nutrition.

Why would this unfortunate situation peak during the young adult years?

It peaks during young adult years because of the laws of natural and sexual selection that have been at work for thousands of generations. These pressures have influenced the modern young woman and young man just like they have influenced countless other species, many of which display similar behaviors during their youth as well.

Let's take the young adult, human male first. For the first two weeks after conception, male and female fetuses are identical. They are both female, which is nature's default setting. At the two-week mark, the XY chromosome starts influencing the creation of and exposure to testosterone, which begins to change the male fetus's anatomy and physiology. All fetuses are also exposed to a certain amount of testosterone and estrogen from the uterine environment. This has a tendency to exert masculinization or feminization influences on the structure and function of the fetus's brain. Therefore, even before we are born, we are all under the influence of sex hormones.

Testosterone: a steroid hormone that stimulates development of male secondary sexual characteristics, produced mainly in the testes, but also in the ovaries and adrenal cortex.

Estrogen: any of a group of steroid hormones that promote the development and maintenance of female characteristics of the body.

Sex hormones literally help create our sexual identity from a universal sex neutral start. David Epstein explains in *The Sports Gene* that it is not possible to create two totally different prototypes for males and females. Therefore, we all start as a female prototype and hormones determine which sex we become over time. That is the reason males retain nipples, even though there is no practical advantage to them.

> One statement I make in my class to bring the point home that our sexuality is irrevocably tied to our hormones is "**Hormones 'R Us.**"

Epstein goes on to say that there are some very good sexual selection-based reasons that young men and young women obtain the physical and mental form that they do (in terms of size, numerical reproductive potential, etc.). They are based, once again, in their requirements to be successful in reproduction. This is true with males of our species as well as with every other species in which the male has more numerical reproductive potential. Males have the propensity to develop to be bigger and stronger than females of the same species and they can create many more offspring than the opposite sex. This is true of human males in that they can inseminate thousands of women over a lifetime if given the chance, while women need a period of approximately one year to produce a baby and return to their reproductive capability. Epstein cites the example of Genghis Khan, who had hundreds of wives and concubines. Through DNA testing, it is now estimated that he alone has male descendants that account for one out of every 200 males on earth. Other DNA research has shown that we have far fewer male ancestors than female ancestors because of males "spreading their wild oats" through prehistory and beyond.[17]

This has set up a situation where humans and other primate males have been selected to compete against other males to be able to mate with as many receptive females as possible. This selection has caused gorilla males to be about twice as large as females and, where possible, to develop harems of four or five females each. Human males are not that much larger than females, but they do have 50 percent more muscle in their lower bodies and 80 percent more muscle in their upper bodies. They also throw better than human females on average. This is thought to have developed when spears and other handheld weapons came into use. It seems that being able to hurt, maim, kill rivals, or at least threaten to do so has been an important part of male sexual selection over the millennia.[18] Steven Pinker writes that over 30 percent of human males were killed by males of other bands during the long hunting and gathering era. The development of agriculture and civilized society has lowered these numbers, but it seems the inclination remains.[19]

The Young and the Reckless

The motivation behind many male raids was the capture of women by the raiding bands. In that world, that meant that some of the men, like the gorillas, ended up with multiple mates, and some with only one, while some ended up with none at all. This scenario had a strong tendency to select for males who were brash, fearless, and yes, reckless.[20] It has been shown by multiple studies worldwide over a variety of different cultures that young males tend to be more impulsive and careless than young females.[21] This innate tendency starts early and really accelerates after puberty. In his book, *Male, Female: the Evolution of Human Sex Differences*, Dr. David Geary writes:

- Boys experience near drowning nearly twice as frequently as girls and die from drowning four times as frequently as girls.
- For each girl that gets seriously burned by fire, three boys sustain similar burns.
- Boys are injured and killed more frequently than girls while riding bikes, on playground equipment, and during sports activities.
- For every girl who is injured on a playground, four boys are.
- Boys experience their highest lifetime levels of testosterone around 17 years old.
- 75 percent of arrests for DUI are males 21-35 years of age.
- Ten times as many men as women are put into prison.
- Over 92 percent of workplace deaths are male.
- Nearly 70 percent of the homeless in the US are men.
- 80 percent of completed suicides are by men.
- Males are much more likely to be both perpetrators and the victims of violent crimes.[22]
- Dating violence is common. Young women between 18-24 years of age experience this most at nearly three times the rate of the general population. Presumably, this is perpetrated mostly by boys and men their own age.
- Over 20 percent of collegiate women experience some form of sexual assault during their college career.
- Sorority members are one of the most highly susceptible groups on campuses.
- Females ages 16-24 are victims of rape at rates that are four times higher than the rest of the women's population.
- Females ages 18-24 suffer the highest rate of rape and sexual assault of all age groups.
- Men killing men occurs thirty-fifty times more often than women killing women.

- Males murdering other males occurs most from ages 18-25 and more frequently in unmarried rather than married men.
- Around two thirds of males killing males results from social conflict rather than crime.
- More than half of these murders are related to status competition.[23]

It is clear that the epicenter for the battles of the sexes for young men is their ability to control themselves. This is true not only in the area of violence, but also their sexuality.

Knowing the influence of our natural and sexual-selection-based ancestral past can be a big help. Some of these tendencies may have been built in. For example, psychologist Dr. Stephan Hamann of Emory University and many other researchers have established through their studies that on average males react more strongly on a neurobiological level to sexual stimuli.[24] These biochemical reactions may have been effective for survival of the fittest and procreation for eons of the past, but they can quickly ruin a young man's life and those around him in our twenty-first century, Western societies based on the rule of law. It can also be very helpful to know that these ancestral conditions have molded young adult men's brain chemistry and structure to cause him to have the tendency to behave in these ways (particularly if he has high levels of testosterone). This will be highlighted and explained further in a later chapter.

In *The Moral Molecule*, Dr. Paul Zak outlines the competitive tradeoff between testosterone and oxytocin (much more on oxytocin later). The upshot of his analysis is that when a man is testosterone-dominant, there are usually challenges in the fidelity department. He points out the fact that young men have twice as much testosterone on average than older men. He goes on to say that one of the results of this is what we have seen often in the news:

"There have been, in fact, so many newsworthy males brought low by their libidos in the past few years that it's hard to keep up. The prize for absolute number of simultaneous affairs goes to golf legend Tiger Woods. The worst name associated with a scandal winner is Anthony Weiner. For shame for audacity, the winner may be former South Carolina governor Mark Sanford, who said he was 'hiking the Appalachian Trail' when he was actually below the equator with his Argentine mistress (then again, Arnold Schwarzenegger having a child with his housekeeper and keeping it a secret from his wife for 10 years—all the while continuing to employ his housekeeper—was arguably, lower still)."[25]

You may say to yourself as you read Zak's comments that many of the men mentioned weren't even young adults, but older men. That is even more distressing news. This testosterone-based snare that many men find themselves enmeshed in is a lasting experience for many. It is not uncommon for men to lose only 1 percent of their testosterone levels per year from age 30 onward.

The other key factor in this sexual compulsion tendency in males, besides the chemistry of the brain, is the architecture of the brain. The amygdala, which is the brain's survival command and control center, is about twice as large in the male brain. Due to its survival-related nature, it is very difficult to turn off when it signals for action to be taken. In males, it is particularly reactive to all kinds of sexual stimuli. As a result, research has shown that sexual stimuli are very difficult for the male brain to suppress or ignore because of these chemical and anatomical factors. This is a monumentally important fact to understand when trying to modify young adult male behavior!

So, the single most threatening challenge young adult men face is what we are identifying as The Testosterone Trap. In all of its related parts—reckless tendencies, violence, and sexual aggression—it clearly revolves around male functions and potential. Again, this is not only characteristic of our species, but many others as well.

We humans, however, have developed a better and more humane way to live and we will try to illustrate how young men can be empowered with self-regulation skills that will enable them to live more successfully within the ethical boundaries of our society. Personally, I've found just knowing and understanding the effects of The Testosterone Trap on me as a man to be empowering and liberating.

Eating for Two in an Inactive, Buffet World

For young adult females, the primary battle faced is also related to their reproductive capacity and function. For young women, the influences of our ancestral past can make life difficult. Having a baby requires approximately 74,000 extra calories above normal metabolic needs for a woman to bring a pregnancy to successful conclusion. Relatedly, we must remember that our ancestral environment was made up of an extreme amount of physical exertion in order to obtain a small amount of edible and digestible calories. It is reasonable to expect that through selection, young adult women's brain chemistry and structure became greatly sensitized to highly palatable food, of which our twenty-first century environment is full. Junk food is readily available, heavily advertised, and in many cases, cheaper than healthier alternatives.

As near back in time as my mother's adolescence in the 1940s, things were dramatically different. She grew up on a farm in southern Oklahoma. Her day started with pumping one hundred gallons of water for the cattle, going to get the cattle on the other end of eighty acres, and bringing them in, currying the horses, gathering the eggs, cleaning the barn, and many other labor-intensive activities. This process was repeated after she and her siblings got home from school as well. Additionally, they had physical education class and sports in school. They were physically active throughout the day on a normal basis. Along with this, they ate mostly the foods they raised on the farm. This included vegetables and fruits, grains, eggs, milk, and fresh meat they had butchered. This was life in a more historically appropriate environment. With this balance, she grew up healthy and was able to have three healthy children.

Seeing that we have come even so recently from such a whole-food-oriented and rigorous past, and keeping in mind the need for extra calories for young women, it is not hard to see the challenge of our twenty-first century situation. Consequently, Dr. Gene-Jack Wang who is the Biomedical Imaging Group Leader at the Brookhaven National Laboratory has discovered that women unconsciously have a harder time saying no to their favorite foods than men. He agrees with the assertion that they have these innate desires because of the ancestral need for extra calories to sustain a pregnancy. It is probably because of this survival-of-the-species-based need for extra calories that a reproductive-age woman's, but not man's, amygdala is very sensitive to and hard to turn off when faced with stimulus from food. This is a female trait that has probably been selected similarly to the way the male trait of a high sexual appetite has been selected.[26]

It is against this background that we remember that the time of greatest increase in obesity happens in people between the ages of 18-25 during the transition from adolescence to adulthood.[27] This is the time period when many go off to college. Physical inactivity, bad dietary choices, increased calorie consumption, increased stress, and disturbed sleep patterns contribute to the rise in obesity during this life stage. This is especially true for college women. Weight gain for college women can be as much as twenty pounds per year, which is substantially higher than their community-dwelling peers of the same age.

College women are exposed to many new experiences and possible lifestyle changes that may contribute to this rise in body fat percentage. These include eating habits, living environment, daily physical activity habits, and increased consumption of alcoholic drinks. Studies have shown that college women report having more stress and lower self-esteem, which may be contributing factors as well.[28]

In regard to energy expenditure, research has shown that some high school senior girls lose half of their energy expenditure between Christmas of their senior year of high school and Christmas of their freshman year of college. Many who were active on high school sports teams (cheerleading, dance teams, marching bands, etc.) become inactive as they move into their college academic careers as many of them were not at the level required to be able to compete on a college team.[29] It is easy to see how this environmental change, both ancestral and the immediate transitional time into college, makes it difficult for young women to stay fit and healthy in the twenty-first century. We have named this syndrome The Female Food Trap. What makes this especially challenging is the time of life in which it is primarily taking place.

Research has also shown that a very high priority of the human brain during young adulthood is mate selection. Many young women are particularly self-conscious about their appearance at this time. As it turns out, there are good, natural and sexual-selection-based reasons behind these unconscious feelings. In *Why Women Need Fat*, William Lassek and Steven Gaulin clarify the ancestral-based reasons behind young women's need to be fit and healthy. They point out that women's waist-to-hip ratio is and always has been important to women's reproductive success. A woman that has a waist about 70 percent the circumference of the hips has the highest probability of having (especially a first) healthy baby. That is because babies produced by women with larger waists[30] tend to be too big to be born naturally through the birth canal. Before the first cesarean section in 1881, these babies, and sometimes their mothers, died in childbirth. In fact, before 1900, one out of every six mothers died in childbirth in the US. Young women with hourglass figures have also been shown to be over three times as fertile as women with larger waists.

Over the thousands of generations of our forbearers, this fact has been burned into the unconscious minds of the males of our species. They cannot tell you consciously why they find an hourglass-shaped female to be so attractive—they just know they do. It is at the level of a primal feeling that is instinctual. Of course, with mate selection, one of the brain's highest goals, this can be problematic living in The Female Food Trap of a college dorm. The lifestyle and the kinds of foods, especially the sweet and starchy ones that women crave, have a tendency, especially in the absence of consistent, vigorous exertion, to deposit excess fat around their waist. This puts them between a rock and a hard place with their desired life outcomes. Just at the time that their romantic life is most important to them, they are struggling to control an addictive food lifestyle that threatens to destroy their self-worth, along with the relationships they so desire. This may be why a 2016 study of 5,455 American adults showed that 35 percent of men are now obese and 5.5 percent are morbidly obese, while 40 percent of women are now obese with 9.9 percent being morbidly obese. It was noted in the report that American women's obesity continues to rise alarmingly.[31]

Overcoming the Battles

A major goal of *Battles of the Sexes* is to help young women and young men understand themselves and each other better in light of the scope of history within the shaping forces of natural and sexual selection. Dr. Peter Gluckman and Dr. Mark Hanson give us a very useful insight into our modern situation in *Mismatch*. They write,

"Just as we inherit both financial opportunities and constraints, so it is that our various pasts—evolutionary and genetic, developmental and epigenetic, environmental, cultural—from long ago and more recent times—create opportunities and constraints on how we can live healthily."[32]

From this knowledge and new insight, young adults will be able to solve their problems and reach their goals (by the way, this is the work of life coaches).

Because of the situation as it has developed historically, we believe that The Female Food Trap and The Testosterone Trap are the biggest immediate challenges for young adults to overcome. The biochemical reactions that fuel both challenges take place on the same reward pathways in the brain. To reiterate once again, because it is such an important insight, it must be kept in mind that a very important factor only recently discovered (that will be explained in even more detail later) is that the structure in the brain that is responsible for survival, the amygdala, responds in concert with the previously mentioned biochemical systems and creates strong female food cravings and male sex cravings. Taken altogether, food issues on average are much more compelling for most young women, while sexual issues are much more compelling for most young men.

To be perfectly clear, we believe that Junk Food and Junk Sex for young adults, especially at this stage of their lives, can be ruinous to their lifetime happiness and health. We are out to make sure that doesn't happen and that they select a mate successfully if they so desire.

Relatedly, there is the Battle Between the Sexes, where many of these issues come together and are synthesized. This forms much of the phenomenon known as sexual conflict, which we will be focusing on in chapters eight and nine, but as an example of the holistic nature of all of these challenges I would like to include an excerpt of my dissertation research that I believe illustrates it.

The qualitative dissertation included ten focus groups and thirty-two in-depth interviews. This is from one of the in-depth interviews. One of our class members, let's call her Angela, was asked if she had taken the Women's Personal Conditioning (WPC) class as freshman and, if so, whether she thought it was helpful in having a successful college experience. Note the interconnectedness of food, male expectations, and body image, and the resulting set-up for sexual conflict in her candid answer:

"In WPC I was not a freshman. I wish I would have been though. Freshman year I slacked off, I was very active, but I didn't worry about what was going on, and relationship wise... I was all over the place. My emotions were high and I didn't worry about myself like I should have. Coach taught us about what we go through. He explained relationships and why we feel the way we feel. I learned about eating habits and nutrition. In my freshman year of college, I barely ate anything. I was always active, and super skinny but never wanted to eat. I was with someone who cheated so I assumed skinny was attractive. I lowered my self-esteem, I focused on what others wanted from me and not about college and what I wanted from myself. If I had taken WPC my freshman year, I honestly would have started to focus. WPC was a wakeup call, not only for a healthy body and eating habits, but for emotional and mental health as well. Girls shared about how guys cheated on them. We all supported one another and pushed each other to do and be better. I could have used that support in my life. I knew how I malnourished my body back in freshman year, but to be honest I didn't realize how

much until WPC. I would definitely qualify as anorexic back then. I would qualify as a woman with low self-esteem. This class really opens you up to who you are and not only what you want out of life, but out of college as well. I think it should be a class you have to take in order to graduate, because whether you walk in thinking you know it all or not, you leave knowing a lot more than you came in knowing, whether you admit it or not."

The remainder of *Battles of the Sexes* will be our best effort to help young adults like Angela to raise their sexual IQ, lower sexual conflict, and gain control of the gender-specific and biochemically compelling voices of destruction in order to be able to navigate the potentially turbulent waters of romance and find a lasting intimacy with the love of their life. We want to, as Plato said, help them learn to find pleasure in the right things despite their ancestral drives. We, as they say, want to empower them to "live romantically, happily ever after."

A SARAH SUMMARY:

- It's as if we've all been transplanted from the Planet of the Past into the Planet of Now, and have become like aliens in our own environment with a poor understanding of how to fit in without being destroyed by our own ignorance.
- For males, an increase in testosterone combined with many decades of natural and sexual selection have developed men that can be rash, reckless, and careless, especially when it comes to relationships.
- For females, more estrogen combined with the same number of decades of natural and sexual selection have developed women that can hardly resist the sugary, fatty food temptations that lay before them daily.
- By increasing our knowledge and understanding of our own and the opposite sex, both The Testosterone Trap and The Female Food Trap can be broken.

Chapter 2

Vicious Cycles:
The Antics of Aunt Flo

"I am particularly concerned about ways in which contemporary reproductive behavior and biology may be a mismatch with the reproductive lives of our ancestors."
DR. WENDA TREVATHAN, *ANCIENT BODIES, MODERN LIVES*

A Battle All Her Own

Before we examine in greater detail the major battles of the sexes in chapters three and four, let's pause for a moment to look at one that women have to fight with their own systems every single month. In my classes, semester after semester, I have made the statement that while men's lives have changed greatly since the Paleolithic era, women's lives have changed *exponentially* over that same time period. That fact has potentially dire consequences for young women. It has only recently been realized that these drastic lifestyle changes could have dramatic effects on women's health.

In *Ancient Bodies, Modern Lives*, Dr. Wenda Trevathan has framed the situation compellingly and logically. She points out that before birth control was invented, women had relatively few menstrual cycles. As pointed out elsewhere in *Battles of the Sexes*, most of their reproductive lives were occupied with being pregnant or breastfeeding. Many of them may have had only 160 menstrual cycles over their entire lifetimes, compared to up to 450 for present day women in Western societies. She concludes that women's reproductive physiology may not be optimally adapted to the routine monthly fluctuations of estrogen and progesterone that happen during a typical menstrual cycle.[33] She quotes reproductive biologist Roger Short, who essentially says that since natural selection has worked over the eons of the past to maximize reproductive potential, women are physiologically ill-suited to spend the majority of their reproductive lives in a non-pregnant state.[34]

A Life Without Tampons

To explain further, the typical life of one of our ancestral women would include having her first period around 16 years old. It would happen this late because her foraging lifestyle would have been so active, and the resulting amounts of food gathered so relatively small, that the body fat build-up required to signal a girl's body to start ovulating would happen much later than it does today. She would have had about three years of non-ovulatory, and therefore non-fertile, cycles and then would have had her first conception around her 19th birthday. This would have been followed by about three years of on-demand breastfeeding. Because of the on-demand breastfeeding and its effect of being a natural birth control mechanism, she would have had her next child about four years later.

Following this pattern, she may have had up to six children with perhaps four of them surviving to reproduce. The final child she may have nursed for four years or more, and this would have taken her into menopause, with the passing of her menstrual cycle barely noticed by her or her husband. In twenty-first century Western nations, this scenario is becoming exceedingly rare. Since the early 1800s, there has been a steady decline in the age at which girls experience their first period. Many of them begin menstruating at age 12 or younger. As a result, many start experimenting sexually and may become pregnant as early teenagers before they are even finished growing themselves. Others use birth control to put off pregnancy until their 30s, 40s, or even altogether.

Breastfeeding and Cancer Prevention

Another difference from ancestral women is that breastfeeding, if undertaken at all, now lasts less than a year. Since breastfeeding is usually not on-demand these days, it does not prevent ovulation from re-starting. Through these methods, many modern women limit their number of children to two or three. This unnatural situation leads to, as noted earlier, modern women experiencing nearly three times as many menstrual cycles as our early ancestors.

During every menstrual cycle, because of the exposure to estrogen and progesterone, cells in the breast and uterus increase their turnover rates in preparation for a possible pregnancy. Each time a cell divides, there is the opportunity for a cancerous mutation to take place. Therefore, these higher cell turnover rates create more chances for mutations. Also, the excessive surges in estrogen impact estrogen-related cancers of the breast, uterus, and ovaries. All of this mismatch with our ancestral environment leads to an estimated rate of breast cancer for modern women that is one hundred times higher than ancestral women or women from present-day foraging populations who don't practice birth control as we do in Western societies. This represents another battle of the sexes that is a result of our cultural mismatch with our genetically encoded biological inheritance. The impact of that mismatch on Western society's women's health and well-being is largely unrecognized and underappreciated. It also, of course, impacts all of those who care about and love those women.[35]

A Word from Sarah

As a woman, I know there is no sense in denying the power of the monthly cycle. It never fails to irritate me when someone asks "Are you about to start?" when I'm reacting more emotionally to certain situations. If you're a woman reading this, you have been asked the same question. If you're a man reading this, you probably know that if and when you ask this of a significant other, you better be prepared with a good set of armor for the response you deserve and should expect from that interaction.

Even though it's irritating as a woman to hear this question, probably because it seems undermining and dismissive of real and true feelings in a given moment, I know it's true. I know I'm acting different.

But why?

Why is it that at some points in a given month I feel strong, capable, put together, efficient, productive, energetic, and downright bada** but other times I feel weak, powerless, flawed, slow, lazy, and depressed?

The monthly cycle is more than just "Aunt Flo" coming to visit once a month. It's a delicate dance of hormones that fluctuate in your body without you even being aware that they dramatically alter your behaviors and emotions. Having a better understanding of this dance of hormones, the general times that they move up and down, and how they can affect the mind and body can help you take back control. It's even

more important for women living in modern societies to un-
derstand this, since as Joe just pointed out, we're suffering
through three times the number of cycles as our ancestors!
But the alternative is having six children and breastfeeding
for thirty years straight, which is just not feasible for most
women today that solo parent, have to return to a workplace
unsupportive of family needs soon after delivering a child,
desire independence and freedom from the responsibility of
children, want to travel the world, have a career that they are
100 percent committed to, etc.

A Hormonal Hell

As Sarah was saying, it is very important for a young woman in Western society to understand the monthly dance of hormones that we call a menstrual cycle. This is especially true when it comes to how it affects their moods and motivations. It should be noted that experts in this area of study believe that one of the causes of some twenty-first century Western women having such hard-hitting premenstrual syndrome (PMS) every month is again the mismatch between our genes that were developed in an environment of heavy exertion paired with a scarce food supply and today's easily obtained, overabundant food supply. This can raise estrogen to supernormal levels, which can cause the extreme hormonal swings that promote PMS symptoms.

In observing my wife over the years, I have witnessed this battle taking place. She was debilitated at times by PMS. I remember coming home more than once and finding her sitting on the couch with the curtains drawn and no lights on and even wearing sun glasses. She informed me that her head was killing her from a migraine headache related to her period, and she couldn't stand any light because it made it worse. Those kinds of scenes have happened for years.

The actual process is described by Dr. Lissa Rankin in *What's Up Down There*. She tells women, every month your body prepares to have a baby. The hormones in your brain pass the word to your ovary that it is time to begin preparing an egg. One fortunate egg becomes a dominant follicle and gets released. The uterus creates a soft, spongy blood nest in preparation for the embryo it hopes to be able to support, and as a result, the lining of the uterus thickens. Once the body discovers that no fertilization has taken place and the woman isn't pregnant, the lining is shed, and that is what we know as menstruation. Then the process starts all over again in the hopes that it might be different in the coming month. This is obviously the very foundation of the life-giving process for humans, and it is to be respected and admired as a feat of nature. It is regrettable, though, that it has to make so many women miserable.

Taming the Madness with Diet

Another aspect of the cycle that can be unpleasant for some women is the ravenous hunger that comes before and during women's periods. In chapter three we are going to explain the relationship between falling estrogen levels and hunger in women, but there is also the compounding challenge of the pre-period hormonal fluctuations that make women more sensitive to their insulin level and how it is affecting their blood sugar levels.

Dr. Rankin provides some natural tips to help women win the battle against PMS. She recommends eating a whole food diet, which means cutting down on processed foods and eliminating elements like caffeine. Instead, she recommends, and I concur, adding more veggies, lean proteins, fruits, whole grains, and healthy fats such as nuts, olive oil, fish, etc. She particularly recommends this for the second half of the cycle. Some women display lactose and gluten intolerance during PMS, so women should be mindful of that as well. Dr. Rankin also recommends managing stress through practices like yoga and taking part in consistent aerobic exercise, which helps regulate hormones. She says that a multivitamin may be beneficial, as well as working with an integrative medicine doctor.[36]

Remember that the purpose of all this commotion is to make it possible for couples to have babies.

An Early Peak

With the change in women's lives regarding professional opportunities, birth control, increased women's rights, and men who, as we'll see, can become hesitant to commit, it is becoming more and more common for women to wait until they are approaching their 40s to start having children. Young women need to know that they reach their peak fertility in their 20s. After that, it can become harder and harder to conceive. By age 45, 87-90 percent of women are infertile.[37] Young women need to keep in mind that their 20s are the easiest time to get pregnant so that they aren't surprised when they have conception challenges in their late 30s.

What are other reasons a woman's cycle is so important?

Every 28 Days

In *28 Days*, Gabrielle Lichterman lays out how women can practically chart their lifestyle by where they are in their cycles. It is pointed out that hormones travel from one organ of the body to another organ through the blood with the purpose of telling that organ to change its action. Knowing how these hormones affect them can help women better self-regulate their behavior and understand their interactions with others as well.

Day one starts with a woman's period beginning. This is when PMS ends. Depression levels drop as the estrogen and serotonin levels they are tied to begin to rise again (more on serotonin later, but for now, it is one of the feel-good hormones). Testosterone levels also begin to rise at this point. This makes women feel more self-assured and assertive.

For the first five days, these factors enable women to feel better and focus more. In the sex department though, surprisingly, these first few days of a woman's cycle can prove to have arousal potential. Congestion in the uterus plus the slow but steady rise in estrogen and testosterone can contribute to this and orgasm is easier to achieve for some women during this time. A potential benefit is that orgasm can relieve cramps by pushing out the menstrual fluid and lowering tension in the uterine muscles, so it's actually recommended. With progesterone gone and estrogen on the rise, women's breasts become less tender and the bloating they were experiencing pre-period begins to go down. These subtle changes continue until around the fifth day when women's periods typically end.

Bow Chicka Wow Wow

The days immediately following the end of their period are when women gradually start feeling their best in almost every way. Sex drive increases as levels of estrogen and testosterone rise, and women typically lubricate at the first sign of arousal. Increasing testosterone levels also make the nipples and clitoris more sensitive. In the next fourteen days, women's thinking changes from more creative and right-brain dominated to more logical and analytical left-brain dominated.[38] Among both married and unmarried people, sex happens most often on day eight of a woman's cycle.[39] As the days move towards day fourteen, rising estrogen and testosterone give women increasing sexual confidence and sexual assertiveness levels. The mounting estrogen levels also raise women's optimism levels.

In the last couple of days before ovulation occurs on day fourteen, women begin to emit higher levels of pheromones. Even though males don't perceive the aromas consciously, they're very attractive to men.[40] Men who are married to women that aren't taking birth control pills (which alter the hormone changes) initiate sex about 30 percent more often around women's ovulation time.[41] Women's orgasms during this time have a powerful, all-over-the-body effect. It is during the time between days thirteen and fifteen that women's sexual desires are directed toward high-testosterone, masculine, dominant guys.[42]

> High testosterone is an indication of a stronger immune system[43], which is important to the health of future offspring and thus is unconsciously attractive to many women, especially around ovulation.

This is the time frame when women are most likely to get pregnant. It seems that instinct has developed over the years to make them desire men with greater genetic fitness when they are most likely to conceive. Let's say a woman is having an affair with a macho, bad boy type. During this time frame, they would typically have more sex with their macho lover than with their own mate.[44]

Day fourteen is a turning point when estrogen and testosterone begin to drop. Women are still near peak levels, so the sexiness continues for a couple more days.

Don't Look at Me. Don't Touch Me.

By day fifteen, with estrogen and testosterone levels starting to decline, a new hormone pops into the scene: noradrenaline. That hormone starts to make women be less optimistic and more edgy. From day sixteen on, libido starts to drop, and instead of opting for sexy clothes, women start going for comfort. The brain makes the determination that the body will not get pregnant this time around.

Women become more introspective and less extroverted. They also start to shift their sexual focus from the macho guy, who might be less dependable and good at being a husband and father, to guys who are lower-testosterone men. These less macho guys often invest much more in being loyal, good husbands and loving fathers.

For the rest of the month, this is the kind of trajectory women's love lives are on. The lessening of estrogen and testosterone also make many women lose some of their body confidence, which has a tendency to lower their levels of extroversion. Rising progesterone levels plug up testosterone receptors in women's brains and make them less interested in sex as the days wind down towards a new period.

On about day twenty, women's brains switch to being more right-brain oriented again. Estrogen and testosterone do start to rise again, but their effects are blunted by the domination of progesterone. This causes women during this phase of the cycle to have a higher need to nurture. This state also decreases the sensitivity of women's nipples and clitoris, causing them to take a very long time to reach orgasm. By day twenty-three, PMS is on the horizon. This can bring on some miserable symptoms for the next several days with increased, ravenous appetite being one of them.

Recipe for the Post-Sex-Pre-Period-Cry-Fest

One silver lining is that sex drive can increase on day twenty-six when the lining of the uterus begins to thicken and bring more blood flow to the vagina. More blood flow to the vagina, whether it is through increased testosterone like earlier in the month or when women think erotic thoughts, kicks the sex drive into gear. As we pointed out earlier, orgasm can help relieve PMS, so women are encouraged to "go for it" during this time of the month. At this point, women are also experiencing withdrawal symptoms like anxiety, weeping, depressed moods, and insecurity. After the low points on day twenty-eight, the cycle starts all over again when women begin a new period.[45]

To Conclude

The menstrual cycle represents an up-down, roller coaster, mood-destabilizing battle of the sexes that women fight every month that most men don't have a clue about. I know that I didn't until the last few years. This is another area where knowledge is power. This vicious cycle and the antics of Aunt Flo need to be taught to both young women *and* young men as they pass through puberty into their reproductive lives. This is another life arena where biological knowledge can give women and men more empathy for each other and help them see we are all in this together.

────────── A SARAH SUMMARY: ──────────

- As a female, if you're not a star on 21 Kids and Counting, then you might be the average twenty-first century woman that intends to have 2.5 kids, more periods than your body cares to handle, continuous tidal waves of hormones, and an increased risk for some cancers.
- Women are no longer living their biological norm, and thus are experiencing unpleasant side effects.
- Understanding how the fluctuations in hormones affect women mentally and physically can help prevent misery through dietary changes and a better awareness of oneself as a woman at different points in the cycle.
- Menstrual cycle in a nutshell:

- Days 1-7: PMS ends, depression subsides, avoid white pants
- Days 8-14: Baby-making, conquer the world time
- Days 15-21: loving cuddles, grab a book and some yoga pants
- Days 22-28: ravenous appetite, ticking time bomb of emotions

Chapter 3

• • • • • • • •

The Female Food Trap
—Junk Food

"Food has replaced sex in my life.
Now I can't even get into my own pants."
MARNIA ROBINSON, *CUPID'S POISONED ARROW*

Our Unique Addictions

I n the late 1990s as I was carrying out work as a fitness professional and personal trainer, I had the new experience of working with a mostly female clientele. Many of these women were in their mid-30s. I noticed right away that most of them were very busy with their jobs, families, and all of their other commitments.

They were so busy that some of them told me they found food had become their main reward system and realized they were addicted, but felt powerless to do anything about it. They could consume it quickly and move on to the next thing that had to be done. Obviously, spending quality time with their husbands and on their love lives had suffered.

I witnessed the phenomenon illustrated by Marnia Robinson's quote at the beginning of the chapter during these years with many young women clients. Food had replaced sex in their lives and, in most cases, had caused them to become overweight. It made me wonder where this had started and if it could be prevented. This curiosity made my switch to working with college students, and eventually mostly college women, very interesting and thought-provoking. I could see that college was where much of women's overcommitted behavior began and started taking notice of sex differences in behavior.

Starting at the university, I had the opportunity to observe some very interesting sex difference phenomena during my years of teaching co-ed personal conditioning to college students. I've always included a segment of the course devoted to covering addictive substances and behaviors. In one lesson, I would take the following addictive substances and display them to the class on the ground through photos: regular and diet sodas, candy bars, cigarettes, coffee, a representation of sexual activity, and simulated cocaine. My first question would be, "Which ones are mind altering?"

Most classes agreed that they all were.

Then, I asked them which were addictive.

Again, most classes agreed that they all were.

Finally, I would ask them to show, in their opinions, which were the hardest hitting and most addictive. This is where things got really interesting. In the co-ed classes, young men invariably rated sexuality highly as a hard-hitting and addictive behavior. Oftentimes it was up near cocaine on the hierarchical rating. But in the women's classes, it was much different.

Frequently, sexual activity was rated much lower by women, often in the neighborhood of coffee, but women rated food at the same high level men rated sexuality. I took note of this in class after class and it rarely varied. I began to see in real life and real time that for young men and young women, the power of food to compel behavior has a significant sex difference. That accidental discovery led me to start studying this phenomenon.

As I started researching, I discovered that Dr. Gene-Jack Wang had found through brain research that a woman's amygdala is less able to turn off craving signals for food,[46] whereas other research showed that the amygdala of young men is more strongly compelled by sexual situations.[47]

The amygdala is the brain's survival, command, and control center and it controls much of our highly motivated behavior, and there are reasons behind a woman's amygdala being shaped as it has been by thousands of generations to react to food stimuli so strongly. Hopefully, after reading and understanding this historical background, it will make more sense to young women and young men.

Reproductive Nutrient Needs

As I continued researching this phenomenon, I became aware of the related work of Dr. Daniel Lieberman, the Edwin M. Lerner II Professor of Biological Sciences at Harvard University. In *The Story of the Human Body,* Dr. Lieberman provides key insights as to why humans, especially adolescent and young adult females, have such a compelling attraction to food.

He describes how humans went through a series of crucial changes over the last two million years, which centered on reproduction and food. The life story of one of our female Paleolithic ancestors was one of a constant search through a hunting and gathering lifestyle for an adequate amount of food for her own bodily needs, for conceiving and carrying a baby to term, and for three years of breastfeeding. A 110-pound woman would require about 1800 calories per day for just her own needs. When she became pregnant or was breastfeeding, she would have needed an extra 500 calories per day. This situation, by the way, would have constituted her lifestyle for most of her adult life.

Our Paleolithic ancestors' biggest challenge was obtaining their daily food by hunting and gathering outside of the tropical jungle environment they had formerly occupied. It required around four miles of walking per day and much labororious gathering to find and oftentimes dig out the foods that were buried underground in the form of tubers. Other dining possibilities were nuts that came in hard shells. There were also berries and roots that were often accompanied by toxins.

Essentially, there was a price to pay for all of those food sources, usually in the form of physical effort.

In these new, open environments with low densities of seasonal, edible plants, the first hunter-gatherers would have had to forage for a large variety of plants. As alluded to earlier, this was oftentimes a very challenging task because of large boulders that might need to be moved, the effort of digging plants up, etc. to get to them. This could take up to twenty minutes of hard labor for each food item obtained. Then, once they were in hand, they had to be pounded or cooked in order to soften the indigestible fiber.

That scenario presented a great challenge, especially to reproductive-age females. Our female Paleolithic ancestor would have probably conceived at about 18 years old and had her first baby at 19 years old. At that time, she would have required the extra 500 calories per day. As the pregnancy went on, she would have become less able to gather an adequate amount of food while still needing the extra calories. Then three years later, she would have become pregnant with child number two. After giving birth, she would be encumbered in her gathering by a toddler as well as the demands of breastfeeding.

Anthropologist Dr. Helen Fisher says that women were responsible for bringing home 60-80 percent of the daily food procurement through their gathering while humans were on the African plains. I would guess that this was probably largely accomplished by the pre-reproductive-age girls and the post-menopausal women who would have not faced the childcare challenges the reproductive-age women did. This childbirth and child-rearing process would have repeated itself and continued until a woman reached menopause. For each of her older children who had been weaned but were not yet able to forage for themselves, she would have needed about 1,000 to 2,000 additional calories per day.

Survival Through Division of Labor

Faced with this situation, it is clear that many of our ancestral grandmothers and their children must have gone hungry and been on the verge of starvation much of the time. This brings us to a key point in our understanding of SEX IQ and sexual empathy. An additional source of food was necessary for reproductive age women and, in order to accomplish this crucial provisioning that was so important to the development of our species, there had to be cooperation between the sexes.

It appears that meat, which is a rich source of calories, fat, salt, zinc, and iron, became part of the human menu about two and a half million years ago. Males, because they were not encumbered by toddlers and didn't have to breastfeed, became the hunters while females gathered plants. This division of labor was a key factor in human success and exceptionalism. Dr. Lieberman writes, "Male chimps rarely if ever share food, and they never share food with their offspring. Hunter-gatherers, however, marry each other and husbands invest heavily in their wives and offspring by provisioning them with food. A male hunter today [from traditional foraging societies in the 21st century] can acquire between 3,000 and 6,000 calories a day—more than enough food to supply his own needs and provision his family... Fathers in turn, frequently depend on plants their mates gather, especially when they come home from a long hunt, hungry and empty-handed."

(Here we remember Helen Fisher's important insight on the crucial nature of women's consistent contribution of gathered, plant-based food to the Paleolithic family dinner table.)

This key, sexually-cooperative relationship made possible the explosive growth of the human brain over the last two million years. In that time, it far surpassed the other mammals' by becoming five times as large proportionally as other mammals and three times as large as the other primates. Large brains are too expensive in terms of energy usage for most species and it would not have been possible for homo sapiens without a nutritional surplus from a sexually empathetic relationship that differentiated them from all of the other animals, and eventually made all great human advances possible.[48]

It should also be noted that it was during this time period that sexual dimorphism (size differences) between the sexes began to lessen. This would indicate a shift away from polygyny and towards monogamy as a mating system, which made romance between a man and a woman start playing a pivotal role in our history.[49] It makes sense that some ancient form of monogamy was a crucial factor in not only the success of the human race but our very survival.

Bottom line: women and men have depended on each other for millions of years and sexual empathy and romance have been a requirement since the dawn of humanity!

Must. Have. Chocolate.

In viewing this historical background, it is easy to see how a female's amygdala could have been genetically encoded over hundreds of thousands of generations to react strongly to food. Especially if that food was readily available, convenient, cheap, and super tasty. Again, this is an appetite that is literally tied to the profoundly important and species-dependent reproductive capability for women.

Introducing the Trifecta

What I'd been seeing in class over the years started making more and more sense. Through the years, I realized that food (and especially the processed and fast food types) posed a greater threat to young women's wellness than it did to young men's. I also realized that three addictive food traps had developed through the decades of processed foods being formulated in labs rather than cooked in kitchens. I knew that these food scientists had formulated concoctions that were intended to make use of the cutting-edge brain biochemistry research that I had been studying since the early 1990s.

I decided I would name them to make it easy for students to remember and apply them in an effort to gain better self-management. Thus, the "**Dopamine Drag**," the "**Serotonin Situation**," and the "**Omega-6 Ordeal**" concepts were born. Once again, I realized that a key point in this insight was the fact that only one of them beckons compellingly to our average young men, while all three are very addictive for women.

1) The Dopamine Drag

In my classes, I've always tried to get across how different the environment that young adults grow up in is compared to that of our ancestors, utilizing the story of my mother and father who grew up on farms in Southern Oklahoma in the 1930s. My mother's day started with hand pumping one hundred gallons of water for the cattle from a steel hand pump on the well, which is very hard labor in itself. Then, she had to bring the livestock in, tend to them, feed the chickens, and gather the eggs. After many more chores, it was finally time to go to school. At school, they had more physical activity by having P.E. class and then came home in the afternoon to repeat many of the morning's chores. They led a mandatorily active life, plus most of what they ate they raised themselves, whether it was food crops or livestock. I gave my students a historical interview assignment for them to complete with their grandparents to illustrate these differences in their own families.

Going back further in time, conditions were even more strenuous and lack of food and periodical starvation more and more commonplace. In those times, if a cave woman or cave man came upon a rotting apple on the ground, it was a major find. The relatively small amount of sugar it contained would have tasted very sweet to them. The sweetness would have also signified that it was probably not poisonous.

We have discovered recently that the dopamine reward system in the brain is tied to a sweet taste in order to drive our ancestors to seek more of the given food, but that reward system today is the heart of the addictive process in humans. Look at some of the sweeteners in today's food. High fructose corn syrup is one hundred times sweeter than the same amount of sugar. Aspartame is 200 times sweeter. I demonstrated the amount of these sweeteners in various popular foods for my classes by passing around vials for them to examine.

Let's just say it's not my most popular lesson, especially with women!

What all this adds up to is that hundreds of millions of people in Western societies are walking around addicted to supernormal sweetness in foods. Soda and other sweetened drinks are the largest single supplier of calories in a US diet and compose 20 percent of the overall total. And diet soda isn't any better. People who drink diet versus regular soda are actually gaining more body fat than the full sugar drinkers because the aspartame (artificial sweetener) only serves to raise dopamine levels. That leads to people seeking other processed, starchy, carbohydrate-loaded foods to complete their food 'high'.

When people drink regular soda, they get their dopamine, serotonin, oxytocin, and, most importantly, their opioids raised. This is the complete high. While they may not seek further supernormally sweet foods, looking for that food high in any form constitutes an addition. We spend a much larger percentage of our lives going around seeking these unconscious highs than we realize.

2) The Serotonin Situation

The next addictive food trap is what I have named the "Serotonin Situation." Women in Western societies run about 50 percent lower on brain serotonin levels than men or women in developing, or foraging, populations.

Those lower serotonin levels have to do with the blood-brain barriers we all have. The blood-brain barrier originally functioned as protection for the brain from poisons, which normally come in larger molecules than non-poisonous substances. But that barrier is causing problems in the twenty-first century, particularly for women. Because of our eating and (lack of) exercise patterns, the blood-brain barrier is now getting clogged up, especially in women, with large-branched, chain amino acids.

In ancient times and presently in foraging populations, the eating and exercise lifestyle takes care of this. The exertion that normally happens (or should) after each meal raises a person's insulin levels and drives the large-branched, chain amino acids into the muscles for repair and building. That is what I classify as good insulin. The good insulin, by clearing the blood-brain barrier, allows the amino acid tryptophan, which serotonin is manufactured from in the brain, to cross the blood-brain barrier. It's worked like that for millions of years.[50]

The problem lies in that most women in Western countries do not eat whole foods or exercise regularly. Their brain levels of serotonin get low, and the symptoms of low serotonin are depression, anxiety, and unfounded anger. In order to raise serotonin levels, the ladies find themselves drinking sodas and eating chips, fries, candy bars, etc. These snack foods cause an insulin spike that clears the blood-brain barrier and allows tryptophan to cross, thus giving them temporary relief. But it also signals the body to store the starchy calories as fat around the waist because the muscles are not working. This situation rings particularly true as women near the end of their cycle each month and estrogen levels plummet (since estrogen levels are tied to serotonin levels in women).

When I ask my classes if they have experienced this, I always see many women's heads nodding. I ask, "How long does the relief last?"

"About 2 hours."

"What happens next?"

"…the snacking begins again."

"And what's the net result of all of this?"

They are usually able to come to the accurate conclusion on their own that the end result is gaining weight around their waists.

I have dubbed this phenomenon "**getting waisted**."

3) The Omega-6 Ordeal

Young women have one more addictive food challenge all to themselves. I call it the "Omega-6 Ordeal." This particular challenge is rooted far back in our ancestral past and is another direct result of the mismatch between our genes, which were molded over the past several million years, and our twenty-first century, Western food environment.

Starting to see a pattern?

The "Omega-6 Ordeal" is directly related to female reproductive functions developed over eons of time. For most of human history, omega-3 fat in our food supply was readily available.

Omega-3 is plentiful in grass.

For most of our history, we ate animals that ate grass.

Grass-fed animals are high in omega-3 fats.

In our modern, Western societies, we eat meat from animals that are raised in feedlots on soybeans and corn. And soybeans are rich in omega-6 fats, but not in omega-3. Also, most of our salad dressings and mayonnaise are full of omega-6, as well as all of the breaded and fried processed foods, whether you get them from a restaurant or the grocery store.

The reproductive connection for young women is in their body's preparation to conceive and carry a child to term, and afterwards to breastfeed for a substantial period. In *Why Women Need Fat*, William Lassek and Stephen Gaulin outline the situation. As girls mature into young women, they are constantly trying to store omega-3 fat on their hips, buttocks, and upper legs.

Why?

Contained within the omega-3 fat is DHA, a major component of a human baby's brain. These stores of fat that nourish future babies are what give many women their hourglass shape (which, by the way, is also why that shape is so unconsciously attractive to young men). Those omega-3 fat stores are used throughout the pregnancy for brain building and especially afterwards as a supply for breastfeeding. For many young women, the time they are breastfeeding is one of the few times in their lives when they can lose size from their lower half. When girls and young women can't get enough omega-3 fat, they just keep craving whatever fat they *can* obtain (even if it's the less healthy omega-6 fat) and proceed to overeat it.

When you pair the Omega-6 Ordeal with the Dopamine Drag and the Serotonin Situation, it adds up to excess fat accumulating on Western young women's waistlines. This can turn into a vicious cycle when it comes to sexual relationships because of the instinctive, unconscious attraction of young men to an hourglass figure.

As I alluded earlier, the hourglass figure attraction comes from tens of thousands of generations of experience with women and children dying in childbirth before the first Cesarean section was performed in 1881. It turns out that if a woman's waist has too much fat around it, the likelihood that the baby's head will be too big to be born naturally through the birth canal rises dramatically. This is especially true if this is the woman's first baby because of vaginal size. Research has also shown that young women with hourglass figures are three times more fertile than those without them.[51] Looking at it positively, it also shows that a smaller waist-to-hip ratio predicts a much greater chance that the baby's head will be small enough to be born naturally.

Nutritionally complicating this further is the fact that many other foods high in omega-3 have mostly disappeared from Western menus. These include foods like cold water fish, flaxseeds and oil, chia seeds, and avocado. When we look at this total situation, we can see why this can clearly be called The Female Food Trap. While men do suffer equally from the Dopamine Drag, women have to face all three every single day. Many women who suffer more intensely from premenstrual syndrome have an even tougher challenge as they approach their period each month with declining estrogen and its linked declining serotonin, causing self-medicating, binge-eating behavior.

With this disheartening, downward spiral, I've also observed many of my female personal training clients replace sex with food in their lives as they enter middle age. For many of them, food became a much more dependable source of pleasure than men over the years. This is one of the major health dangers we want to help prevent in their future!

Reflections from a Student

The other thing that makes it so easy for many young women to allow junk food to replace sex in their lives is that it is so easily available beginning in college. I got this letter from a former student, let's call her Sidney, that described her and so many other college women's freshman year junk food experience:

"To understand why I even registered for a wellness class in the spring of my freshman year, you would have to know about my fall semester. I came to MTSU fresh outta high school where I worked two jobs and spent the majority of my time outdoors in the country. I lived half an hour from the nearest town and lived between three family farms. To eat at a restaurant or grab fast food was a luxury.

"Being a freshman living in the dorms on campus, it was mandated that I have a meal plan. I was able to eat anytime at the cafeteria-styled buffets or grab fast food from the KUC and Cyber Café. Coffee and snacks just needed a swipe of my card and they were mine for the taking. I went from having 'whatever is in the fridge' options to endless (and effortless) options at my fingertips—literally I could order a pizza and have it delivered to my dorm, paid for by Flexbucks!

"I gained 15 pounds in four short months. I remember going home for the Christmas holiday and my grandmother saying she didn't even recognize me. Before returning back to Murfreesboro for my spring semester, I managed to lose 10 pounds by simply eating three square meals a day like I had before.

"But it took Coach's wellness class to help me become healthy again. I thought I would be learning how to run or lift weights properly. I did learn that but I also learned things like why my body would crave salt or sugar, how to make simple substitutions in the foods I ate, which parts

of my brain were impacted by foods and relationships, how being outside could improve my mood and how to live with ENTHUSIASM! Unlike the books and articles I had read in the past, Coach's class gave me advice I had to pass on. I made lifelong friends that I still talk to today. I work out each week doing both aerobic and anaerobic exercises I learned through the class.

"I am now a senior in college and can honestly say I have learned more applicable life lessons in a one credit class than any three-credit class I've taken thus far. It helped the transition to college significantly and has impacted my eating, thinking and exercising."

College Female Food Trap

Sidney's story of a vastly different lifestyle as a young woman at home as opposed to college is far too common. That is one of the reasons I chose to create the Women's Personal Conditioning (WPC) class. I wanted to see if more comfortable and effective college P.E. environments could be created for college women.

As I mentioned briefly in the Introduction, in the years leading up to this time I became aware of some very interesting, emerging research regarding the pivotal, societal role of young women's wellness. In this regard, recent scientific breakthroughs have made abundantly clear the importance of helping girls and young women on a population-wide level get a handle on The Female Food Trap. An entire new medical discipline has been created by the discovery that conditions in the human womb, as a fetus is being carried, have strong effects on the health of the future baby and child all the way through adulthood. This new field is called Developmental Origins of Health and Disease (DOHaD).

The scientists of DOHaD have discovered that either undernutrition or overnutrition of females can predispose their children to heart disease, diabetes, and osteoporosis as adults. The nutritional environment of the womb is created as a girl (a future mother, if you will) grows up and becomes a young woman. If the right amounts of muscle, fat, vitamins, and minerals are in place from living a healthy and active lifestyle, the fetus has the chance to optimally and healthfully build all of its vital organs. If not, then flaws are built into at least some of those vital organs, such as the heart, kidneys, lungs, etc.

In short, the diets and body compositions of today's girls and young women will largely determine the health of the next generation and can even affect the one to follow. For example, some of the DOHaD researchers have reported that two-thirds of adult-onset diabetes could be eliminated in in a single generation by employing effective, preventive health promotion initiatives to improve the health status of girls and young women across Western societies.[52]

It made me feel great when some of the young women from the Women's Personal Conditioning focus groups showed that the DOHaD science had impacted them. Here is a comment from one of those women:

"The discussions about how our health state affects our future family helped motivate me."

Now we just have to get those DOHaD insights out to young women worldwide so they can take informed action to change the health trajectories of themselves and their future families.

So *you* and *your* partner can take informed action to change the health trajectories of yourselves and your future families.

A Word from Sarah: One Fish, Two Fish, Red Fish, Blue Fish

Whenever I picture a village from way back in the day, I picture the village set alongside a river, stream, lake, or other body of water. It's impossible to live without water, so it wouldn't have made sense to take residence somewhere without an abundant supply of it. Since water and fish go hand-in-hand, it would be safe to assume that our biology as we know it today is dependent on the nutrients that fish and other water-dwelling life provides. But there can be some barriers to eating an adequate amount of fish nowadays.

First of all, you have to know what to buy. The production of fish through farming has compromised its nutrient quality similar to the way the production of other meats has.

Second, you have to know how to cook it. We've all been there. We plan a nice meal, spend one to two hours preparing and cooking, and at the end of all the toil and labor, end up with dry and overcooked (or raw and undercooked) fish or other meat, vegetables that were seasoned inappropriately, rice that we put too much water in, etc., not to mention a disaster of a kitchen and a sink full of dishes to wash, and we end up throwing a pizza in the oven anyways. Fish has never been easy for me to cook. If you have the time and resources to take a cooking class, it would serve you (and your family and friends) abundantly well throughout your lifetime. Of all the basic necessities of life, food is the one that requires the most skill, and a cooking class or even cookbook would be a fantastic use of time and money.

Third, you need to eat fish at least twice a week to reap the most benefits. This is where planning your meals ahead of time comes in. If you lack a plan, odds are you may not end up consuming an adequate amount of omega-3 fats in your overall diet.

Some foods that contain omega-3 fats include: fatty fish (Salmon, Tuna, Trout), shellfish (Crab, Mussels, Oysters), Oils (Walnut Oil, Canola Oil, Flaxseed Oil), Nuts and Seeds (Walnuts, Chia Seeds, Flaxseeds).

What's for dinner?

Besides living next to water with an abundant supply of fish, the purpose of our ancestor's daily work was centered around how and what they would eat and feed their families. Today, planning to eat is an afterthought at best. We know where our food comes from—the grocery store or restaurant— and we eat whatever we can get our hands on, whenever we can get our hands on it.

Where has this eating behavior led us?

As a society, we have become a people burdened with self-induced sickness, often referred to as chronic disease. Diabetes, high blood pressure, heart disease, kidney failure, cancer, and obesity are affecting us by the droves when we have the power as a society to prevent much of it.

So what do we do about it?

What are we supposed to be eating?

The Dieter's Dilemma

This is a loaded question. The film What the Health would argue we should all be vegan. If you dabble in Crossfit, you may find yourself on the paleo train. If you have heart disease, someone in the hospital probably "educated" you with a handout about the D.A.S.H diet. If you had twenty pounds to lose in a month, you may have had a friend suggest a keto diet.

If you're a baby boomer with extra time on your hands, you're hanging out in weekly Weight Watchers meetings. If you're a trendy hipster, you probably eat "clean." (What does "clean eating" even mean? Run your food through the dishwasher before you eat it?)

You get the idea. There are a million different diet strokes for a million different types of folks. Besides, new "research" comes out at least weekly it seems, telling us that we should be avoiding this and eating more of that, only to find out a year or two later that the recommendation is the total opposite. Nobody in the realm of nutrition research can really make up their mind about effective diets and "optimal" foods.

Nutrition research is flawed.

First of all, it is often funded by whoever has the most money. Second, correlation is not always related to causation. Just because people that eat more eggs have higher cholesterol (correlation) does not necessarily mean that the eggs themselves have caused the cholesterol to rise (causation). The way news sources spin the research will always have you believe that A causes B when it's just frankly untrue and entirely misleading. The misinformation put out by media about food research gridlocks the average consumer into inaction based on confusion.

Three Wise Words

I counsel clients on nutrition education as a part of my work with my business, Simpletic Nutrition. I stay far, far away from "diets" because they don't work long term. This is difficult because people generally want a prescription for a magical diet that will solve all weight woes in a jiffy.

(Do a Google search of all the past Biggest Loser winners

and see how many of them kept the weight off through crash di-
eting. Spoiler for those without access to Google: none of them.)

There is definitely one piece of advice that I feel confident
giving to nearly everyone I come in contact with regardless of
their health goals.

Eat living food.

Strip away all of the flawed nutrition research, the thou-
sands of diets out there, and all of the documentaries, books,
magazine articles, etc. It all comes down to the fact that hu-
mans thrive when they eat living food. I'm a self-proclaimed
nutritionist with a minimalist twist, and it can't get more min-
imal than those three words. You could even strip it down to
*two words: **Eat Life**. This principle, without needing any fur-*
ther education on nutrition, can help make food decisions in
nearly every scenario. There is no more "bad versus good" or
"healthy versus unhealthy" when it comes to food. It's either
alive, dead, or somewhere in between. You should be eating a
majority of your foods from living sources. By that definition,
if 51 percent of the foods you eat are alive, you're on the right
track. Never expect that you would be able to eat 100 percent
living foods 100 percent of the time. There is a space in life for
the enjoyment of foods that you would have considered "bad"
foods. A pack of candy on Halloween, a piece of cake at a
birthday party, pecan pie at Thanksgiving, chocolates on Val-
entine's day, a cocktail at a bachelorette party. These are some
of life's sweet joys. They are not "bad" or "unhealthy"—but
all of those do fall on the spectrum of being dead, so they are
not foods you would want as part of your daily eating routine.

The Countertop Test

I'm going to give some examples of what I mean by living

and dead foods for the sake of full clarification.

First example: Hamburger. Choice 1: Grass fed ground beef hamburger patty purchased at your local grocery store and cooked on a grill in your backyard. Choice 2: McDonald's hamburger. Place both on a countertop and see which one spoils. You'll find that the McDonald's hamburger won't spoil nearly as quickly as your backyard grilled hamburger. Why is this? Preservatives, salt, and artificial chemicals. McDonald's burgers are already dead, so how could they spoil? Things don't die twice. If you consider whether or not a food will spoil on a countertop if left out for a period of time, this can help tell you whether or not it is alive.

Second example: Apple. Choice 1: Hostess Apple Fruit Pie. Choice 2: Apple and peanut butter. Which snack has veins? Yes, I mean like the ones in your own body. Look reeeeally close at the apple next time you eat it. Which snack required sun, water, and soil to grow? Which snack turns brown and begins to spoil within minutes of being sliced in half? Which snack has seeds? It's easy to see here which snack contains living food.

Life Begets Life

Now consider your own eating routine. How often are you eating living foods versus dead foods? It is not uncommon for someone to go days and weeks without consuming a living food. They wake up to Pecan Wheels and coffee for breakfast, head to the local fast food restaurant for a burger and fries for lunch, and finish the day with a store-bought pizza with ice cream. A human being cannot eat like that for years and live a healthy life—it simply isn't possible—and we're seeing a scenario of early, preventable death by chronic dis-

ease playing itself out in the Western world. How much bet-
ter could that same person thrive if the day began with eggs,
strawberries, and oatmeal, lunch consisted of a large salad
heaping with seasonable vegetables, diced chicken, walnuts,
sunflower seeds, mandarin oranges, and vinaigrette, and the
day finished off with salmon, asparagus, and a sweet potato?

Life begets life.

When you focus your meals on filling your body with liv-
ing foods, your body's health and energy will reflect that focus.

Understanding Your Cravings

When you find yourself in the inevitable situation prior to
the start of a new cycle, when your cravings are stronger and
your willpower is weaker, knowing how to swap the lesser op-
timal food cravings out for living, nutrition-packed alternatives
will leave you feeling more energetic and, perhaps, a bit lighter.
See the table below for some craving swap suggestions.

Craving	Why I'm Craving It	Swap
Ice Cream Chocolate	High Fat, High Carbohydrate	Avocado on Whole Grain Toast Sliced Apple or Banana and Nut Butter Fresh Fruit Smoothie with Greek Yogurt Sweet Potato with Teaspoon of Butter Homemade Sweet Potato Fries Dark Chocolate Covered Almonds Trail Mix
French Fries Potato Chips Pizza	High Fat, High Salt, High Carbohydrate	Handful of Honey Roasted Peanuts Edamame in Soy Sauce Homemade Potato Soup Veggie Pizza on Cauliflower Crust Whole Grain Bagel with Cream Cheese Rice Cake Salmon and Baked Potato
Candy	High Carbohydrate	Grapes Blueberries Strawberries Raspberries Fresh Peach Mandarin Oranges Raisins, Dried Apple Chips

Beside these few simple swap suggestions, I will leave you with a few extra tips to help with controlling cravings and beating The Female Food Trap for good.

1. *Always have a plan for meals and snacks.*
2. *Eat three to six meals daily around the same time.*
3. *Eat your most substantial meal of the day either one hour prior to exercise, or in the hour immediately following exercise.*
4. *Avoid telling yourself you can NEVER have a certain food, such as chocolate. Indulge mindfully, and in small doses, when hunger is not at its peak.*
5. *Exercise daily to release the feel-good hormones that you may be seeking through food.*
6. *Drink twelve ounces of water when a craving hits to both curb your appetite and ensure you're staying hydrated.*
7. *Be mindful of coffee and alcohol consumption, especially during this time. Coffee can increase your craving for sweets, and alcohol lessens your willpower.*

A SARAH SUMMARY:

*   Food can prove to be more addictive for women due to the difference in the female versus the male amygdala.

Chapter 4

• • • • • • • •

The Testosterone Trap
—Junk Sex

"Lust is temporary, romance can be nice, but love is the most important thing of all. Because without love, lust and romance will always be short-lived."
DANIELLE STEEL

The Young and the Restless

In my experience, many young women wonder why many young men are more interested in "hooking up" than they are in creating a romance that will develop into more than a short-lived relationship. They are looking for "the love of their lives" and expect men to have the same motivations.

(Danielle Steel, among many other authors, has even created an extraordinary career selling romance novels to women who desire this destiny *because* that motivation is so strong.)

Eventually, many young women, after being traumatized by relationship after relationship through no fault of their own, come to the conclusion that all young men are dogs (and many much more colorful names) and that men are motivated only by their loins. Young adult men are often accused of letting that appendage below their waists rule their every thought and action when, in reality, it's their brains that rule the day (and especially the night).

Now ladies, before you begin thinking of this revelation as an "I told you so" affirmation of your long-held suspicions, let us be clear: just like women, men are influenced by the chemistry of their brains, which in turn influences the chemistry and actions of the rest of their anatomy.

It probably comes as no surprise to you at this point that the male brain has two and half times more space than the female brain devoted to sexual drive and has a larger brain center for action and aggression. This means sexual thoughts run through a man's mind far more frequently than they do a woman's.[53] A man's brain chemistry creates a craving for new sexual experiences the same way an addict's brain craves cocaine or heroin. Its main ingredient, dopamine, plays a major role in motivation and reward, surging before and during a pleasurable activity like sex. This makes men want to repeat a behavior, especially one so crucial to the survival of the species.

I am sure that some of the early sex researchers like the pioneering Alfred Kinsey wondered what was up with what they were seeing in their experiments with animals. He took note all the way back at the start of his research in the 1940s that a male rat could not be distracted during intercourse by cheese crumbs but that his female sex partner could.[54] Again, the extra food is more critical to the young female rat's survival and reproduction than to the males because of the extra caloric requirements of pregnancy. Evidently, human males and females are not the only mammals that have to deal with sex differences in levels of compulsion toward junk food and junk sex.

Advances in neuroimaging have allowed current researchers a peek inside the human brain, providing the opportunity to document how the brain's reward system can get hijacked by certain pleasures, causing it to continuously thirst for more while inhibitory control centers experience a failure.

Chemistry 101

Now before you ladies accuse of us of giving men an excuse to run amuck with their desires, let's walk through the cerebral chemistry that leaves so many young adult men open to temptation with some common brain chemical culprits and the chemical reactions they cause.

1. Testosterone: While both genders secrete testosterone, men can have up to 183 times more total testosterone than women. This is the hormone that gives guys their swagger. This is also the chemical that makes them exhibit animalistic aggressive behavior like screaming "KILL HIM!" at the TV during a football game, or gives them the desire to hop on a motorcycle and enjoy a little wind in their helmetless hair.

2. Dopamine: The brain's pleasure predictor and transmitter. Stoked by novelty, risk, and newness, Dopamine can produce quite a high. It is what makes you excitable and talkative. It makes your heart race and speeds up your pulse. Dopamine is also essential for our survival and happiness and when dopamine is in short supply or really jacked up in men, it can cause a lot of problems.

3. Serotonin: Think of it as the "happy chemical." Serotonin maintains well-being by calming anxiety and relieving depression. It affects mood, sex drive, appetite, anger levels,

memory, and sleep patterns. Serotonin is known as the master neurotransmitter since it affects many of the other neurotransmitters in the body.

4. Adrenaline: Adrenaline revs men up! The term "fight or flight" is often used to describe the circumstances under which adrenaline is released into the body. Spiked during highly stressful and physically exhilarating situations, think of adrenaline as the brain's warning system. It allows better coping with dangerous and unexpected situations. When adrenaline is teamed with testosterone, look out!

5. Vasopressin/Oxytocin: All of us are familiar with the notion that male dogs pee on their territory to mark it. Vasopressin works much the same way. During sexual activity, vasopressin and oxytocin being released into the brain reinforces the bond between partners. These hormones are even thought to induce males to become aggressive towards other males—particularly those who come near what's theirs, if you know what I mean. And while all this male protectiveness and territoriality may sound sexy to some, keep in mind that it doesn't alleviate the pull towards territory that other men are standing guard over. After all, "he who dies with the most toys (or conquests) wins!"

6. Prolactin: In women, prolactin increases during pregnancy, which stimulates the production of breast milk. In men, prolactin sends them into a fetal-positioned nap after doing the deed. Also known as the refractory period, higher levels of prolactin shut down a man's interest in sex, allowing him a recovery period until the next "go around."

7. Opioids: Opioids play into the whole pleasure and reward balance. You know that "runner's high" people talk about? That is the result of naturally-produced chemicals called

endogenous opioids, also known as anandamide. These are the brain's painkillers. They lessen our perception of painful nerve signals, protecting us from fully feeling them with an effect known as antinociception.[55]

The chemistry of lust is similar across the board throughout the animal kingdom. What sets humans apart is our ability to override what chemistry begs us to do.

DoN'T Do It Like They Do on the Discovery Channel

Our large cerebral cortex helps us be rational, yet can also leave us prone to unconscious temptations. Although we already know we *can* make healthier choices and self-direct our path, that isn't always what happens. Perhaps it would behoove us to first understand our potential internal struggles by looking at how monogamous relationships, particularly marriage, reached the precarious state they're in today, and what we can all do to protect and keep our home lives harmonious.

Portrait of the Western Family

In the last three decades in particular, the portrait of the family has seriously shifted. Less than half of American families are still intact (with the original mother and father together). Many children are growing up in homes with a single head of household, oftentimes just the mom. Households also now can include unmarried parents living together and step families that become "blended" through divorce and remarriage. Not to mention that the rate of divorce seems to go up exponentially with each marriage. According to the US Census Bureau, 41 percent of first marriages, 60 percent of second marriages, and 73 percent of third marriages end in divorce.[56]

The picture becomes even bleaker when looked at from a basic chemical level. The "hot and sexy" chemicals (like dopamine) drop for a married man, yet they rise, along with oxytocin, for a married woman within a good relationship. Bluntly put, the chemicals that result in a reward high need to be stoked up within marriages. As we've already learned, danger and newness are the greatest triggers for revving up dopamine and its chemical wingman, testosterone. So unless your male partner can find a creative way to harness and ignite this chemical current, temptation will be difficult to resist.

Thrill Ride Gone Wrong

Men who have been pulled towards adulterous behavior, like Tiger Woods, are engaging merely for the high or the thrill of the conquest, not for love. I am sure you've seen Elin Nordegren Woods. You must realize cheating doesn't have much to do with the beauty (or lack thereof) of the wife. It's the different (new) woman, and with her the new experience that spikes the dopamine and provides the temporary new thrill. That dopamine can bring the heights of pleasure to a peak experience. Located in the nucleus accumbens, a collection of neurons within the brain's striatum, dopamine is thought to play a role in reward, pleasure, laughter, addiction, and aggression. Whether it's a lustful or loving act that occurs during a sexual encounter, a strong mix of chemical changes increases the levels of serotonin, vasopressin, oxytocin, and endogenous opioids swimming around the brain, causing the body to relax and take in pleasure, as well as inducing bonding with one's partner. It's a frightening and intoxicating scenario.[57]

But there are more factors than chemistry we need to take into account. Let's not forget what that large cerebral cortex does for us. It helps us process cultural and social factors. It gives us the ability to decide another course, whether that is avoiding the temptation of promiscuous sex or the bottle or diving in headfirst. We do learn from and become conditioned by our social experiences. It could be the reason why some people tend to gravitate towards the same type of partner again and again.

So, how do we take this chemical state, and all its genetic and environmental influences, and make love a long-term attachment, which offers stability to our children?

Little House on the Prairie

Scientists think they may have found the answer in prairie voles.

A very social critter, prairie voles are among a small portion of mammal species that appears capable of forming monogamous relationships. They bond and pair for life after a marathon twenty-four-hour mating session. Preferring to spend time together, they actually avoid meeting other potential mates. They groom each other and participate in nesting for hours. The males aggressively guard their partners, and when their pups are born, both genders are loving and attentive parents.

The prairie vole's cousin, the montane vole, on the other hand, is a player with no interest in long-term partnerships. This cad of a vole seems to enjoy playing the field by indulging in its own version of hookups. The most intriguing thing about the behavior differences in these vole cousins is that it's the result of just a few genes. Genetically, these voles are 99 percent alike!

Just two little hormones make all the difference.

The monogamous prairie vole experiences a release of oxytocin and vasopressin during sex, unlike the montane vole on its quest for hookups. Remember that these chemicals feed the bond between partners during sexual acts and cause them to be protective of their territory. If these hormones are blocked, the prairie voles seem to join the "dark side" with their montane cousins, embracing infidelity.

Interestingly, if they're given an injection of oxytocin or vasopressin, but kept from having sex, the prairie voles still form a preference for their chosen partner. What's even more fascinating is that when these hormones were injected into the montane, it made absolutely no difference. The montane vole was still a player. The reason behind their difference in reaction is that the prairie vole has *receptors* for oxytocin and vasopressin in the brain regions associated with reward and reinforcement, while the montane vole does not. This begs the question of whether humans, another member of the exclusive club of potentially monogamous mammals, have brains that are similar to prairie voles.

Researchers in social attachment at Emory University have been striving to answer this question. They explain that the brain's reward system is designed to make the voles, as well as other species, do what they should do: sleep, drink, eat, and have sex. Without this reward system, animals might forget basic upkeep, which could lead to the end of the species. Animals continue to rest, have sex, and nourish themselves because these acts feel good and release dopamine into the brain. It should be noted that the female prairie vole experiences a 50 percent dopamine increase in her brain when she mates, something definitely worth sticking around for![58]

Porn Culture

Now before we start injecting men with extra oxytocin and vasopressin, let's not forget there other factors at work as we move through society. Advertising, skimpy fashions, and the constant input of the world we live in have bent our natural systems out of shape.[59] Imagine what this does, particularly in a male brain, which is more susceptible to visual stimuli than a female's.

Once again, the amygdala, the survival command and control center of the brain, is the main catalyst of reaction and it is very difficult for young men to consciously override being tempted by sexual situations.[60] For thousands and thousands of years, males have reacted on their survival-based emotion centers in order to have the best chance of passing their genes along to future generations. And recent research shows that for perhaps those same reasons, the amygdala is the most powerfully reactive, motivational structure in the human brain. This fact alone could explain the popularity of pornography in the male population!

While love and the laws of attraction can be explained and vividly illustrated chemically, we can't forget that in the end, humans still have the choice of embracing a healthier lifestyle. For many high-testosterone young men, this means they must not simply walk away from temptation—they must run!

Points to Remember

If any of you guys need motivation to safeguard your relationship with the love of your life, you may wish to consider these points:

- Married men are 250 percent less likely to die prematurely than divorced men (from any cause).
- Married men have better immune systems.
- Married men are less likely to commit suicide; they also report lower levels of depression and stress.
- Married men are less likely to commit murder.[61]

Why does having a spouse mean such a boon to a man's physical and mental well-being?

First of all, the extremely large oxytocin boost from having a steady, trustworthy companion is *immense*. The accompanying rise in serotonin is also quite beneficial. We also have to take into consideration that women act as motivators for men to take care of themselves by keeping up with medical screenings, going to the doctor when there are perceived medical problems, regular dental visits, etc.

Finally, in keeping with the theme of this book and especially this chapter, being in a committed, romantic relationship substantially lowers men's serum testosterone levels. If children come along as a result of the relationship, it lowers them even more. This seems to be one of nature's long-term solutions to the hankering of men for Junk Sex and the life-wrecking destructiveness of The Testosterone Trap.[62]

In *Wild Sex*, Dr. Carin Bondar, an expert in the area of animal sexuality, puts it this way:

> "For me, one of the most fascinating things about human sexuality is our adherence to sexual and social monogamy. Almost no other mammals exhibit such a strategy for valid biological reasons. Where did monogamy begin? Why did it catch on so completely in our species? While there is an abundance of research on the topic, I am unsure as to whether there is one overriding conclusion. Although it may not be 'what all the other animals are doing', I am still a believer in the notion of a monogamous relationship. I think that this is because while our bodies may want to, our brains don't allow for it. The complex suite of emotions that accompanies any sexual relationship lends itself to having one partner (or one preferred partner) over being highly promiscuous."[63]

We strongly agree with Dr. Bondar's assessment and assert that based on the scientific evidence, monogomy is especially challenging for human males, but is also highly possible with the right life circumstances. Through education and the resulting intentionality, young men can learn, as Danielle Steel says, that love, and not just lust, is the most important thing of all and it can lead to a lifetime of happiness, health, and prosperity!

——————————— A SARAH SUMMARY: ———————————

- A man's brain chemistry creates cravings for new sexual experiences in the same way that an addict's brain chemistry craves heroin.
- What sets us apart from animals is the ability to override those cravings.
- Men who succeed in monogamous relationships are set up for a healthier, longer life.

PART II

Human Sexual Chemistry

Chapter 5

. . . .

The Chemical Laws of Attraction—Secret Sex Signals

"Human's greatest problem today is not to understand and exploit the physical environment, but to understand and govern their own conduct."
FRANK A. BEACH, THE FATHER OF ENDOCRINOLOGY

Much of the romantic world is controlled by forces that cannot be seen and work at the level of the unconscious mind. That is one of the factors that makes human sexuality so challenging to control. We must keep in mind that the unconscious part of the brain, generally the limbic system, is stronger when it comes to motivation and drive than the rational part of the brain, the cerebral cortex.[64] The limbic system is literally at the center of the brain and simply has more outputs, both to the cerebral cortex above and the brain stem below. While the cerebral cortex is the rational part, the brain stem controls automatic functions like breathing, digestion, blinking, etc.

Pheromones: His Favorite Perfume

The limbic system is what determines how we feel. It's like a Boeing 777 being controlled by the cockpit—such a large object is being controlled by such a small part of the airplane, just like the limbic system in the human body. It often takes a lot of overt effort for the rational control center—the frontal part of the cerebral cortex—to override compelling impulses coming from the limbic system, generally represented by electrical and chemical reactions happening within the brain that are communicated to the rest of the body. Sometimes, these chemical reactions are a response to internal stimuli, and sometimes they are a response to external stimuli.

When it comes to sexual attraction, pheromones are a major source of external stimuli. These chemicals are often airborne, and when we inhale into our nasal areas, we cannot actually smell them but rather only perceive the message they are sending to our unconscious minds. Women in particular send out these signals, and they align with their menstrual cycles.

One of the most famous research projects in the recent past was one that dealt with comparative earnings of female strippers and exotic dancers. For those who were not on hormonal birth control, their earnings rose sharply when they were in the fertile window of their menstrual cycle. It was discovered that hormonal birth control lowered the amount of pheromones released during the fertile window because the women's bodies were constantly being told by their internal chemistry that they were already pregnant. Therefore, the olfactory systems of the male customers were not stimulated to create the chemical reaction in the limbic system that ignites attraction.[65]

The specific type of pheromone that females release is a group called copulins. Copulins are made of fatty acids that are in female's vaginas throughout the month, but migrate towards the opening at the times of highest fertility. From there, they become airborne and strongly affect men, especially men that are in close proximity (such as when receiving a lap dance). They can then travel to the vomeronasal organ high inside the nose.[66] Women can also be strongly affected by men's pheromones, which are linked to the level of androgens (like testosterone) in their sweat.[67]

Another interesting pheromone study is one in which men with symmetrical features and those with asymmetrical features were told to wear the same shirt for a week. A random sample of women were asked to sniff the shirts (once they were off the men) and determine if some were more attractive than others. The ones worn by men with symmetrical features were chosen over the ones of men with asymmetrical features.[68] Somehow men's body odors have been linked over thousands of generations to their genetic fitness. It was also found that females have a keener sense of smell than males. For women more than men, the right bodily smell can be a deal maker or a deal breaker.

Ovulatory Cycle: Humans in Heat

Recent research shows that for women who are not on hormonal birth control, their menstrual cycle has a strong effect on their sex drives.[69] Again, the first five days of their cycle are made up of their menses, or commonly named period. At this time, estrogen, testosterone, and progesterone levels are all low. Testosterone levels are at their lowest on day twenty-four and gradually rise until day fourteen, at which time they begin to decline slowly. Even though testosterone levels are relatively low during menstruation, women may feel higher levels of arousal because of the lining of the endometrium thickening.

From day seven to fourteen, testosterone and estrogen levels are continuously rising. This causes women to experience many changes. Their faces actually become more symmetrical and attractive.[70] Their lips thicken and their skin clears up.[71] Thinking becomes sharper and quicker. Women have a tendency to dress more provocatively during this time,[72] and be both more sexually guarded and sexually motivated. They report having more fear of being sexually assaulted or raped during this time by undesired assailants, and have a tendency to do less walking unaccompanied or in darkened areas.[73] At the same time, there is an increase in their motivation to seek genetically higher-quality mating opportunities. They are more drawn to masculine, symmetrical faces and bodies and deeper voices.[74] If a sexual liaison does occur, they have less of a tendency to use birth control. Therefore, the chance of becoming pregnant during one of these trysts is increased. This may also be influenced by the fact that women are more likely to reach climax in one of these liaisons than normally.[75]

In summary, once again, if a married woman is going to cheat, the chances are that it will be around the time of ovulation and with someone that is of higher genetic quality than her husband. In order to prevent this, it is important that women become aware of this unconscious phenomenon and tendency.

Circadian Hormone Rhythms

An additional area that adds to the drama of this hormonal interplay between women and men is the circadian rhythm we all have. This rhythm of timed hormone secretion is tied to the twenty-four-hour light and dark cycle provided by the sun.

If you think about it, every other creature on this earth has the same relationship with the sun cycle and lives in harmony with it naturally. We are the only species that fights it with impunity. That is why we have such a hard time when we travel across time zones rapidly—the sudden change in the sun's relation to our internal clocks. Our bodies like regularity. And one aspect of our circadian rhythm that women should be especially aware of is that men's testosterone levels, along with their cortisol levels, are highest in the morning. This means that men may be more sexually motivated during that time of day than any other,[76] which can be problematic if his job begins early and he's heading out to work in this state. Women's hormonal fluctuations, as we have discussed, are more closely tied to their monthly cycles. They do not have a peak hormonal secretion in the mornings as do men and oftentimes their proclivity for sex is actually stronger in the afternoons or evenings.

With all this hormonal and circadian rhythm disparity, it's no wonder sexual conflict so easily occurs even with high levels of attraction.

A SARAH SUMMARY:

- We are driven mostly by our unconscious mind through the limbic system of the brain, which requires continuous and effortful taming by the cerebral cortex.
- Female copulins are pheromones that trigger attraction in the limbic system of men through the vomeronasal organ in the nose.
- Male androgens are pheromones that strongly affect a woman's attraction to a man.
- Especially around day 14 of a woman's cycle, her body and mind are gearing up for the potential to reproduce in ways she's not even aware; men are waiting, and ready, at the dawn of each new day.

Chapter 6

· · · · · · · ·

The Visual Laws of Attraction

"Pretty woman, walking down the street.
Pretty woman, the kind I like to meet."
ROY ORBISON

Eye of a Tiger

M en are much more visually aroused by sexual stimuli than women since their brain anatomy is significantly different from women's.

There is a part of the brain called the medial preoptic nuclei77 of the hypothalamus that is over two times as large in males as it is in females. As its name hints, it is located in the middle of the limbic system, situated at the point where the optic chiasm transmits visual pattern impulses from the eyes. It is here that what we see enters the brain and is inserted into the hypothalamus, and the hypothalamus is one of the most important areas of the brain when it comes to motivation. The medial preoptic nuclei are also sensitized by testosterone, which the male brain contains much more of than the female's.

Women's brains have an analogous structure, but the medial preoptic nuclei is much smaller. Instead, a female's analogous structure is the ventromedial hypothalamic nuclei, which is located behind the medial preoptic nuclei,[77] further away from the optic chiasm, and therefore less influenced by vision. This area processes feelings of love, lust, and appetite for food in females. It's not that visual sexual attraction isn't a factor for women, but it is simply stronger for men. Proof of this can be found in places such as the pornography industry, where the majority of material is created for male viewers (Studies have shown that the smaller percentage of women that do like porn actually prefer the same type of subject matter as the guys. Porn with male actors and models is viewed primarily by gay men).

Men's visual preferences have been finely tuned over thousands of generations. This is true especially when it comes to women's waist-hip ratio. Social scientists over the years thought that each culture had its own pattern of what was considered attractive, and that those body-shape fashions come and go. They thought that society dictated what was considered attractive to their young people. Then a researcher named Dr. David Singh in the early 1990s wondered if there might be a deeper connection between a woman's body shape and her health, and that if such a connection existed, if it might make certain female shapes attractive universally across cultural lines. That would mean that attractiveness was not a matter of fashion, but was hard wired into men's brains.[78]

Another researcher, David Buss, was doing related research at about the same time, looking at human's sexual preferences in thirty-seven different cultures worldwide. He found that women were most attracted to men with high social standing and plentiful resources. Men, on the other hand, in all thirty-seven cultures, put more emphasis on youth and physical attractiveness. Surprisingly, media exposure, or lack thereof, didn't seem to have any effect.[79]

36-24-36—It's Science

Again, it turns out that a woman's waist-hip ratio is not only a good indicator of her health, but is also a strong anatomical indicator of her potential fertility. The hormone that helps produce a small waist in relationship to the hips is estrogen. And estrogen is also a crucial hormone for a woman to become pregnant and determines where fat is deposited in her body. Therefore, lower waist-hip ratios signify health and fertility.

By the time a young woman is an older teenager, she typically has a .72 waist-hip ratio. In other words, her waist is 72 percent of her hips. Women in porn magazines like Playboy were found to have a waist-hip ratio of .67, or their waists are 67 percent of their hips, which is much smaller. Dr. Singh then did a different experiment where men were shown drawings of women of varying sizes and waist-hip ratios. No matter what the *overall* size of the women, men preferred the lowest waist-hip ratios. The size (as in total bodily volume) didn't seem to matter as much as the waist-hip ratio did (up to a point).[80] That confirms that it is not so much weight that determines women's attractiveness to men, but shape.

Sir Mix-A-Lot must have really done his measurement research for *Baby Got Back*. He was spot on the .67 ratio found in porn magazines.

Interestingly, Dr. David Bainbridge of Cambridge University showed that women have even higher expectations of their figures than men do. One study showed that men prefer women with a body mass index of 18.8, a .73 waist-hip ratio, and a .69 waist-bust ratio of. Women, on the other hand, were slightly less demanding of themselves in the overall size department with a preferred body mass index of 18.9, but tougher on themselves with a preferred .70 hip-waist ratio and a preferred .67 waist-bust ratio.[81] It seems that when it comes to their own body expectations, women can be very demanding.

Meanwhile, other social scientists who were out to prove that Dr. Singh was wrong about a universal preferred waist-hip ratio set out to replicate the study with males from other countries and cultures around the world. With only one exception (Tanzania), the men all preferred the lowest waist-hip ratio.

What could be driving this preference in men worldwide for women with low waist-hip ratios?

It turns out that it is a matter of natural and sexual selection, and therefore a matter of biology.

Baby Got Back... and DHA

Remember in *Why Women Need Fat*, William Lassek and Steven Gaulin showcase research that points out that docosahexaenoic acid (DHA) is crucial in the formation of the human brain?

One third of the typical brain is made of this fatty acid. DHA happens to be one of the main components of omega-3 fat, which is stored primarily in the legs, buttocks, and hips of young women. These areas act as reservoirs of the critical nutrient.

DHA is also crucial in the creation of human baby's brains, especially in the last trimester of pregnancy and during the course of breastfeeding.[82] This may seem simple, quaint, and outdated, but it is a pivotal component of human success, and yes, has even impacted our very survival as a species. Once again, for the vast majority of the past two million years, our hunter-gatherer ancestors had to struggle to make this work under opposite conditions than those of the twenty-first century, developed world. Instead of having a ready abundance of food-like products low in nutrients but high in calories, our ancestors had to scrap, scrape, and labor to find and procure rudimentary nutrition. These coarse, fiber-filled, primitive, vegetable-derived foods were not only moderately nutrient-dense in many cases, but they were also very scarce and low in calories.

In *The Story of the Human Body*, Dr. Daniel Lieberman describes this situation well. Gathering food was very challenging for our ancestors because they had to walk at least four miles a day just to find a few edible, underground roots, berries that were defended by toxins and nuts that were encased in hard shells, amongst other edible foliage. This, by the way, is why humans don't naturally want to exercise on their own. Being able to relax when not having to exert brought energy, balance, and health in ancient times and so that tendency to relax when given the opportunity was selected for. Clearly, because of the cultural mismatch, this is not an advantage to our health today.

It Didn't Come Easy

When our ancestors went out gathering food, there were always challenges. A single root could take twenty minutes to extract and often involved moving large rocks, tree branches, etc. That single root would then have to be pounded or cooked before it was even digestible. Plant foods, especially non-domesticated ones, are high in non-digestible fiber and relatively low in nutrient density. Two million years ago, early human women were caught in a dilemma completely opposite of the conundrum women face today. A young woman who weighed 110 pounds back then would have needed about 1,800 calories per day just for her own body's basic function and would have required an additional 500 calories per day if she was pregnant or nursing. Most of a young woman's life was spent pregnant or nursing, so for the majority of her adult life, she needed 2,300 calories per day. As time went on, she would also need 1,000-

2,000 additional calories for each of her older children who could not yet forage independently. Studies of present-day hunter-gatherers show that mothers who are nursing or encumbered by toddlers cannot get near their needed 2,300 calories. That means women must have faced a near perpetual state of starvation much of the time during our ancestral mothers' lives.

A Word from Sarah

As a woman that has just ended a forty-month span of nearly continuous pregnancy and/or breastfeeding, I can 100 percent confirm those caloric need estimates. I experienced a tremendous increase in appetite while pregnant and nursing and could eat unimaginable amounts of food. I used to serve as a food service manager, and would often eat the same foods that the residents in my facility ate every day.

I could pile so much food on a plate that the staff couldn't help but give me the most astounded looks. Like the emoji with the wide eyes. They were always asking how I stayed "skinny" eating like that—I can tell you, eating for two, and a few times three (breastfeeding while pregnant), definitely doesn't hurt! I had to ensure that I was balancing the increase in calorie consumption with regular, almost-daily moderate to intense physical activity. I was running 5K races at five months pregnant with my first, and strength training has remained an important aspect of my routine throughout my childbearing years. Staying active daily in those ways has not only helped me maintain an ideal weight despite my appetite, but has also been an effective stress reliever (a lifesaver for a full-time working mom!).

Forever Eating for Two

The increased calorie needs during pregnancy and breastfeeding set up a situation where women are genetically encoded to seek calories when and where they can find them. Sweetened foods are one of the strongest motivational stimulators, *especially* for human females. Our brains have been encoded to recognize these kinds of foods (or food-like substances) as calorie-dense nutrients. Therefore, modern-day women have a predisposition for those kinds of foods and are driven to overeating them when they are readily available.

Again, solutions to our ancestral, near-starvation situation would have had to include pair bonding (monogamy) with men who, unencumbered by young ones, could hunt for meat and provide those extra calories. Hunting for meat started at least 2.6 million years ago. Meat is nutrient- and calorie-dense. It is a rich food source in many other ways as well, carrying significant amounts of zinc and iron.

Hunting most likely started out more as scavenging because it took a long time for projectile weapons to be invented. It is unlikely that women who were pregnant, nursing, or taking care of toddlers could scavenge or hunt much, which produced a natural division of labor in which the men hunted and the women gathered. Food sharing would be practiced between these human couples, which again was crucial for the human brain to have the energy to enlarge. Male chimps, in contrast, do not usually share food with their offspring. It is the human pair-bonding phenomenon that allowed humans to become the extraordinary species they have. Over the last two million years, the human brain has doubled in size, becoming proportionally three times the size of other primates and five times the size of other mammals.

On days when the hunters were unsuccessful, the women's gathering of plants was critical to stave off starvation. As Dr. Lieberman says, "It is hard to imagine how they could have survived without both females and males provisioning each other and cooperating in many ways."

Our proportionally enormous brains most likely developed over the ice age to help our species deal with different geographies that we were driven into. We needed to be able to think, analyze, remember, and develop many other complicated cognitive exercises. Much of the expansion was probably used to negotiate increasingly complex social relationships and cooperative endeavors that became our human hallmark trait. It took a surplus of energy to accomplish this, which was only provided by the conditions we have just described: cooperation between a man and a woman.[83]

All of this relates back to why those reservoirs of omega-3s on women's hips, buttocks, and thighs are so important to reproduction and, therefore, so unconsciously attractive to men.

But why are small waists on women in combination with full hips and legs so important (and tantalizing to men worldwide)?

Mechanics of Birth

The answer to that question lies in the mechanics of the birth process. If a baby is born naturally, especially if it's the first birth for a woman, it cannot be too large to fit through the birth canal and young women's waist sizes are correlated with the size of their babies. The bigger the waist size of the woman, the larger the baby. Therefore, it has been genetically encoded into men's unconscious minds that a woman with an hourglass figure has a good chance of delivering a healthy baby the first time. In fact, studies have shown that young women with hourglass figures are three times as fertile as women with a larger waist and are much more likely to be able to deliver a healthy baby naturally.

As we have seen, women in our ancestral past struggled to get enough food energy to achieve the lower body DHA stores, so there was rarely a problem with women having too large of a waist. With our twenty-first century women, the challenge is the opposite. Because American women eat mostly grain, grain-fed animals, soy-based dressings, and foods fried in soy, they have an abundance of omega-6 and a comparatively small amount of omega-3 fat in their diets. This means that American women's percentage of DHA in their fat is lower than women's in other countries and ancestral women's. The lower the percentage of DHA in a woman's fat, the more body fat she needs to achieve the same total DHA of the non-American women. For example, if she is getting half the amount of DHA in her diet, she will need to have twice the amount of body fat in order to store the same overall amount of DHA. With the lower amount of omega-3 in their diets, American young women may be storing up to two times as much fat on their bodies in order to achieve the required amount of DHA reserves. That situation is then counter-productive because it creates larger waist sizes and forces women to carry excess weight.[84]

It is a complex scenario that has great impact on relationships. It affects both those between men and women and between women and food.

Symmetry

Understanding our ancestral past is pivotal for creating healthy bodies and healthy relationships in the twenty-first century. For men, physical attractiveness is a deal maker or breaker. Dr. David Geary illustrates studies that show that men desire facial features that indicate sexual maturity, but, at the same time, relative youth. They also place a high amount of emphasis on symmetrical body and facial features and proportionally longer legs in women. They like breasts to be larger than average and to be symmetrical as well. In particular, men prefer facial features that include large eyes, prominent cheekbones, and a bigger than average smile area.

A larger section of men's brains lit up when viewing attractive women's faces than average in studies. Men also seem to be more easily motivated to act on those feelings, especially when their testosterone levels are high.

Women too prefer physical attractiveness, just not as strongly as men do. They are more attracted to men who are taller than average, have an athletic but not too unnaturally large muscular body, which would include about .8-.9 waist-hip ratio and a .7 waist-chest ratio. In other words, they like a moderately-muscular V-shape in men. Facial features that they prefer are similar to those men prefer. They like larger than average eyes, prominent chin and cheek bone structure, and facial symmetry.

Beauty in the Eye of the Beholder

As noted earlier in our discussion of pheromones, women's preferences during the fertile window of their menstrual cycles seem to focus on different aspects of male characteristics than during other times of their cycle. During the fertile window, they become more attentive to attractive men and may be more easily aroused by sexually explicit material. They are also more attracted to taller men and to the scents of men with symmetrical body features. Men with masculine faces and voices are more of a turn on during this time as well. They are drawn to men who exhibit dominant behavior and personality traits, as well as high creativity. This is true especially if a woman is paired with a long-term mate who does not possess these exemplary masculine characteristics. This can sometimes be the case with so-called trophy wives, who may have been more influenced by a man's monetary holdings at the time she decided to marry him and only later started having these types of thoughts and impulses.

During the low fertility part of her cycle, a woman's preference for these "macho" physical and behavioral characteristics declines, and her preference for men that exhibit emotional sensitivity and fatherly tendencies increases.

Additionally, both sexes prefer clear skin tone and bright eyes. These traits are more pronounced around the time of ovulation in women. One other thing that is attractive to both men and women is dilated pupils. When looking into the face, particularly the eyes, of someone we are attracted to, our pupils unconsciously dilate, as if wanting to take in more of the beautiful sight.[85]

It seems it's true then that beauty really is in the eye of the beholder.

--------------- A SARAH SUMMARY: ---------------

- Men are far more visually aroused by sexual stimuli than women due to a significant difference in brain chemistry and anatomy.
- Men all over the world, from all societies, and with all different environmental influences are attracted to women with low waist-hip ratios.
- A low waist-hip ratio signifies youthfulness, optimal health, fertility, and optimal DHA levels for successful reproduction.
- Both sexes are more attracted to the opposite sex with overall symmetrical features, but women tend to factor in social standing and a sense of security more than men.

Chapter 7

• • • • • • • •

The Female Sexual Mystique

*"Literature is mostly about having sex and
not much about having children.
Life is the other way around."*
DAVID LODGE

Female Choice

Study after study has shown that women are pickier when
consenting to mate than men. In the world of science, this
phenomenon is called **female choice** and it has been making
the difference for women in areas such as available nutrition,
protection, genetic quality of their children, and paternal investment
for at least two million years. In his study across thirty-seven cultures,
psychologist Dr. David Buss documented that one of the highest
priorities that women have in terms of long-term mate qualities is the
ability to procure resources. Again, during the Paleolithic, this could
mean the difference between life and death. Related traits in a young,

up-and-coming potential mate would be qualities like ambition, work ethic, social status, IQ, emotional maturity, and chronological age.

While there are certainly benefits that come with those characteristics, there's also a challenge. A man with those aggressive acquisition characteristics may also be inclined to seek casual sex with many different women. In other words, their willingness and ability to commit may be lacking. That puts a high priority on men who have all of the above characteristics, but are also sincere and can show acts of love directed at just *one* woman.

On the other hand, for our female ancestors, having the love and commitment of a man who could be pushed around by other men physically would have been a mixed blessing. Women who mated with smaller, non-physical men would have never had security from other men. Men during the Paleolithic who were taller, athletic, and equipped with a muscular build could give their wives protection from animals, as well as other men who acted like animals. The women who selected men based on their ability for physical protection had a better chance of surviving and producing children. The desire for this type of man was (and is) genetically encoded in women, even though societal conditions have changed today.

Even if a man manages to have all of the above characteristics, if he gets sick or passes away, he is no longer able to team with a woman to produce a family. Therefore, potential husbands are also judged on their health status and long-term health prospects. Women in the study of thirty-seven cultures said that good health in men was anywhere from important to indispensable in a mate. Markers for this, again, are symmetrical faces and bodies and higher masculinity. Asymmetrical features show mistakes the body made in self-construction. These may be evidence of other errors the body has made in systems such as the immune system. It turns out that symmetrical men have fewer illnesses than asymmetrical men over their lifetimes, and men that are masculine also signal that they have good physical health. Men with bigger, lower jaws, pronounced brow ridges, deeper voices, and V-shaped torsos show development during adolescence that was influenced by major amounts of testosterone. However, too much testosterone can be bad for men's health in the long run. Only men with strong immune systems can afford to carry that testosterone load for long periods of time. Men with weaker immune systems unconsciously cut back on testosterone production.

On the topic of masculine men, women find them especially attractive for sexual flings. By using that strategy, they can maintain their relationship with their perhaps less masculine but wealthy husband and still garner the benefits of the more genetically fit hunk. Those benefits might include having sons who, because they too eventually become hunks, would have a better chance of siring many children themselves. This is called the **sexy son hypothesis**.[86]

The Mystical Total Package

With all of the male classifications outlined above, there are still more important traits that women consider crucial. Men with high testosterone are known to be more aggressive and violent. A man with all of the above qualities who is cruel or mean can prove to be impossible to live with. So, women also desire men who are intelligent, dependable, and emotionally stable. These are the men who make good fathers and husbands. Research shows that there is a correlation between intelligence and men who value exclusive sexual relationships (interestingly, women showed no such correlation between intelligence and desire for exclusive relationships).[87] Men who have the combination of high testosterone and high intelligence are rare commodities indeed!

In summary, it's easy to see why the question of what a woman wants in a man can be so puzzling for men. It can definitely constitute a mystique.

And yet, with our ancestral history, it is easy to begin to understand why women's preferences can be so complex and have so many variations. Their preferences are very dependent upon context and there are facets that are being analyzed (consciously and unconsciously) on many different levels. Their decisions reflect innate programs that are the result of the challenging survival situations that ancestral women had to deal with over millions of years of female choice.[88]

Testosterone and Oxytocin

There is a trade-off between testosterone and oxytocin. Higher levels of testosterone drive down levels of oxytocin and vice versa. Generally, men have many, many times higher levels of testosterone than women and women have substantially more oxytocin (and estrogen that boosts its effect) than men. That's why women on average are more empathetic, more focused on the well-being of others, more generous with money, time, and volunteering, and are overall, more charitable than males.

As we have said before, The Testosterone Trap is also a major influence in the tendency of men to be players. But at the same time, testosterone gives men the tendency to be judgmental of other men who practice infidelity. Elliot Spitzer, a former New York state attorney general, was famous for crusading against corruption, while at the same time patronizing prostitutes from an escort service. During the 1990s, some of the top congressional leaders who were adamant about impeaching Bill Clinton because of his connection to the affair with Monica Lewinsky were also carrying on. Before it was over, each of the five, family-values Republicans were revealed as being involved in their own adulterous affairs and at least one had fathered an illegitimate baby by an affair.

In both of the above cases, males display less empathy than females. Testosterone actually blocks the binding of oxytocin to the receptor, which lowers men's empathetic responses and also affects their willingness to do the understanding or virtuous thing. The higher the testosterone level, the more oxytocin is blunted, and the less empathy men have. The less empathy someone feels, the less generous they are. So, testosterone particularly interferes with the uptake of oxytocin, essentially throwing a wet blanket on the tendency to be caring and feeling.[89]

I have witnessed this phenomenon many times in my classes. Each semester we do what we call a campus food tour to check out the nutrition quality of the food that is offered across campus. In all my years of doing this learning activity, I have never observed a male offer to come to the aid of a classmate who wasn't able to do the running associated with doing this tour. It has, however, been commonplace for women who realize that their injured classmates would not be able to keep up with the running group to request that they be allowed to walk and accompany their injured classmate so their classmate doesn't have to be isolated from the group.

Each time I've observed this phenomenon, I have examined the situation carefully to see if the requesting young woman is asking just to get out of running. Each time, it has been an athletic student who loves physical activity and is a leader in the class. As I've continued observing, I've become convinced that it is all about the empathy she is feeling for her classmate who isn't able to fully participate, as well as empathy for her unwanted state of debilitation. She is willing to forgo her own workout in order to ease the loneliness and stress her friend is feeling. I believe it is a sterling example of what we are discussing here with the magnified effects of the sex differences when it comes to testosterone and oxytocin ratios in young men versus young women.

Risky Business

Too much testosterone and too little oxytocin also make young men society's greatest risk takers, such as high-risk investments. A famous example that Dr. Paul Zak uses in *The Moral Molecule* to illustrate this is the Donner party wagon train back in the 1800s. The men in the party chose to stake their fortunes on an unproven shortcut. As many people know, that supposedly quicker route got them into the Sierra Mountains later in the season than advisable, which got them stuck in the snow of what we now call Donner Pass. About half of them died and the others had to turn to cannibalism to survive. Records of personal accounts show that the women in the Donner Party had been strongly opposed to taking the unproven trail.

Oftentimes, indeed, mother knows best. Women are more risk averse in many areas of life. Research shows that they carry more life insurance, are safer drivers, and prefer to invest their retirement funds more conservatively than men. This, once again, reflects the higher level of oxytocin and lower level of testosterone.

Cyclical Preference Changes

Although they generally do have a lower level of testosterone than men, remember that one time that testosterone does rise and peak in women is just before ovulation. This makes women more sexually driven and, particularly, more driven to connect with masculine, dominant men with high quality genes during that time. Higher levels of testosterone make both genders less willing to trust. Around ovulation, women become less willing to trust their security in less safe situations. They are more unconsciously aware that they have greater vulnerability to becoming impregnated by an unwanted partner through sexual assault during this time, so they take counter measures to avoid it. In other words, women are more sexually driven, but since they are also more likely to get pregnant they aren't, as men may be, simply more promiscuous with just anybody; they are only more promiscuous in a focused way with more masculine, genetically superior hunks whose baby their unconscious minds are motivated to carry.

Testosterone and Stress

In the stress of normal daily life, the oxytocin and testosterone levels help women be better equipped to deal with our twenty-first century society. Under moderate stress, women have the tendency to come together and support each other. The researcher who discovered this, Dr. Shelley Taylor, called it "Tending and Befriending."

In males, more testosterone is secreted under stress, and they generally have an angry and fighting response, which proves to be negative for men's long-term blood pressure and health.

Another place high testosterone in men makes them different than women is their ineptitude in picking up social cues. Studies have shown that people with high testosterone levels spend much less time making eye contact than lower testosterone people. This means that many men miss the social information they could be picking up from reading eye contact. In many cases, men come across as aloof and uncaring, which is read as being emotionally absent in their interactions with women. By not putting enough emphasis on empathy and intuitive perceptions, men miss out on the important communications of eye contact, voice inflection, body language, and social context, which doesn't go unnoticed by women.[90]

An Orgasmic Paradox

In addition to what has been outlined already about the differences between the sexes, young women should understand the finer points of the development of their sexuality. If you are a young lady reading this, you probably already know that your sexuality is quite different from your man's.

For one thing, you have probably noticed that he reaches orgasm every time you make love, but you don't always get there. And when you do, it takes much more effort to achieve than it does for him. This is especially true during the last half of your menstrual cycle. Being educated about what has happened in the development of our species can help you understand what may be going on. The research of Masters and Johnson shows that nearly all women, if they are sufficiently prepared and stimulated, reach orgasms, but oftentimes it takes more than intercourse alone. Research shows that only about one fourth of women are orgasmic from intercourse alone; it usually requires manual or oral stimulation of the clitoris.

There seems to be a paradox in human sexuality.

There is a mismatch between the male of the species, that has an orgasm and ejaculates easily and quickly, especially if he is younger, but then is impotent for a considerable time afterwards, and women of the species, who are definitely capable of multiple orgasms with no period of impotency.

This too could be seen as a part of the female sexual mystique.

Masters and Johnson's research shows that human females, like some other primates, have the biological machinery to get into a state of high arousal and stay there for an extended period of time given the right circumstances. In *The Woman that Never Evolved*, Sarah Blaffer Hrdy says, "In the human female, orgasm may be greatly facilitated by high arousal prior to intromission [intercourse], and women, unlike men, do not return to a physiologically unaroused state after orgasm, but to the pre-orgasmic period."[91]

What kind of physiological behavior could leave this kind of biological mechanism as a legacy in modern women?

Dr. Mary Jane Sherfey, an early sex researcher and feminist, hypothesized that this female sexual response and multiple orgasmic capability came from our deep ancestral past. She says that with no cultural restrictions, primate females like chimpanzees and bonobos have sex between twenty and fifty times per day during the height of their heat. These will usually include several acts of sexual intercourse in rapid succession with different partners. This behavior provides the reproductive advantage of almost certain pregnancy and the advantage would be accomplished by females with the most insatiable sexual appetites. That trait would then be selected for in later generations since those females would have achieved pregnancy the most.[92]

Until the last part of the twentieth century, in view of the difficulty many women have achieving orgasm, the clitoris was looked upon as a poor comparison to the penis as far as efficiency goes. It was seen as the reason why women's inability to climax could be so problematic. Further research showed, however, that women have a larger network of excitable erectile tissue on the inside, and that the clitoris is just the tip of the iceberg. It is, in fact, a much more substantial area than is represented in males. It also works in a complementary fashion to males by the vagina enlarging, or what they call "tenting," while at the same time self-lubricating. It is definitely a wondrous physiological feat that, in tandem with men's physiological feat of erections, have made the miracle of human reproduction possible for millions of years.

In *Read my Lips*, Dr. Debby Herbenick and Dr. Vanessa Schick cite more recent research by Dr. Helen O'Connell that shows there are different parts of the clitoris that work together to enlarge during sexual arousal and mysteriously become part of women's orgasmic process. This research supports the assertion that females have a larger network of internal erectile tissue connected to the clitoris that cannot be seen. It seems that the vagina, clitoris, and urethra all move together when any of the individual parts are stimulated. Dr. O'Connell suggests that these surrounding synergistic organs be renamed the clitoral complex. I believe that would help many people, especially men, to better understand and appreciate the complex process that goes on during female sexual arousal.[93]

It has been concluded by some that the challenge of human female orgasm achievement compared to men's relatively easy and automatic response is not the clitoris itself, but the *type* of sexual activity undertaken. Dr. Sherfey asserted that the woman was not inadequate or inferior sexually. If liberated from cultural restrictions, she could practice her sexuality like some of the other primates do. She could have sex all day long, day after day, with one male after another, until she is physically exhausted.[94]

Obviously, human culture restricts this type of behavior and, for at least the last two million years, pair-bonding between human males and females has been one of the most important factors in our extraordinary development as a species.

It seems that we may have switched back and forth several times between different mating systems during deep prehistoric time, but for about the last four million years, we have been moving from a moderately polygynous form of relationship to a more romantic, monogamous one. As a matter of fact, during those last four million years, having a pair-bonding drive seems to have been selected for in women and became a major reinforcer of monogamy in our species. Recent research has shown that after sex both men and women experience surges in testosterone and oxytocin. But, and this is a very big but, men secrete much greater amounts of testosterone, which actually blocks their oxytocin receptors and dampens the post-sex bonding drive that women are experiencing. This promotes the tendency for them to have the attitude that they have been there and done that and are ready to move on without any further commitment. It may explain why some men leave women waitng to hear from them again after a casual sexual encounter and instead "ghost" them in our current hookup culture. We believe this biochemical phenomenon in men runs against women's best interests and hookup culture is definitely a negative for many twenty-first century women.[95]

I did want you young women reading this book to know about this sexuality paradox phenomenon so maybe you could understand yourself, your emotions and feelings, your sexuality, and how your body works better. Your wonderfully complex sexual desires, responses, and physiology should make more sense to you now that you understand the differing developmental periods our species has gone through to arrive where we are today.

Alcohol Differences

One other phenomenon with potentially crucial consequences that young women should be made aware of is the different effect that alcohol has on them compared to men. Alcohol actually increases testosterone levels in women, while it decreases them in men. This means that women can become much more sexually reckless if they are drinking, especially if they are drinking during the particularly fertile window of their menstrual cycle (days nine to fourteen).[96] It leads to scenarios where young women wake up after a night of drinking and ask: I did what? With whom? Where?

Also, studies show that around 64 percent, or nearly two thirds, of college sexual assaults included alcohol as a factor.[97] We want women to be aware, safe, and in control of their faculties at all times, recognizing that alcohol makes them more inclined to make risky decisions than it does men.

In conclusion, we have to remember that all of these genetically-encoded chemical reactions and related behavioral inclinations were selected for in the *vastly* different environment of the Paleolithic era. The lesson here is that by using the knowledge of these reactions and inclinations, we can employ our conscious minds to make choices more suited to our success in our modern, twenty-first century environment.

―――――――――――― A SARAH SUMMARY: ――――――――――――

- Women want men that are symmetrical, masculine (but not too masculine), intelligent, muscular (but not too muscular), healthy, dependable, emotionally stable (but not too sensitive). Clear as mud?

- Men with very high testosterone, while attractive to women (especially around the time of ovulation), suffer from lack of empathy, understanding, caring, and feeling, and tend to participate in riskier behaviors.

- The female requires more stimulation to reach orgasm, but once reached, doesn't experience a period of impotency (as males do), and is capable of multiple orgasms (as males are not), showcasing a physical sexual mismatch.

- Women may become far more promiscuous and sexually reckless when alcohol is used, as it increases testosterone levels. Alcohol use in men actually lowers testosterone. Alcohol consumption during the ovulatory period by women should be done cautiously.

PART III

. . . . . .

The Battle Between the Sexes

Chapter 8

• • • • • • • •

The Battle Between the Sexes: Sexual Conflict

"In the battle between the sexes, men and women will go
practically to the end of the earth in illogical, irrational
ways to give each other pain."
KAREN DeCROW

A Bug's Life

What is behind this battle between the sexes?

It is the sexual conflict that arises because each sex has mating strategies that differ from those of the other sex.

Each one's optimal reproductive fitness is best served by their particular strategies and does not necessarily take into consideration what is best for the other sex. Let me give you an example from the insect kingdom. Have you ever heard of a praying mantis? The female praying mantis is famous for literally biting the head off of its mate as they are having sex.[98] She not only gets inseminated in the process, but she also gets a meal, which ups her chances of being in a positive nutritional state to produce healthy offspring. Of course, this doesn't do much for the well-being of her mate, but reproductive fitness in nature is not about the well-being of the couple, but instead about the well-being of each individual sex.

Another insect, the fruit fly, may be the most researched species when it comes to sexual conflict. It too is very illustrative of each sex's concern for their own well-being. It turns out that fruit fly semen contains a chemical that has the effect of an anti-aphrodisiac on the female. At the same time, the semen contains chemicals that increase egg production in the female and put the sperm of other males out of commission. These sperm competition chemicals have an additional effect that is similar to spider venom and can shorten the female's lifespan. This cocktail of chemicals has been selected for the reproductive fitness benefit of the male only, because the male's reproductive interest in the female is for only one copulation. Her reduced lifespan means nothing to him on a reproductive level because it won't be his semen the next time. The amount of his genes in the future gene pool will actually be proportionally raised by preventing her from mating with future males. Therefore, this set of genes and traits has been selected for in the male.[99] The female fruit fly, in turn, evolved defenses against the toxicity in the male's semen.[100] When traits in one sex harm the reproductive fitness of the opposite sex and there is selection in that sex to counterbalance the harm, it's called sexually antagonistic coevolution. This kind of sexual arms race is very common throughout the insect and animal kingdom.

When it comes to human sexual conflict, there have been developments on a multitude of levels. In "Human Sexual Conflict from Molecules to Culture," Dr. Gregory Gorelik and Dr. Todd Shackelford point out many of these arenas.

Sea Men

Let's start by looking at semen. Human semen contains chemicals that manipulate females' physiological and psychological mechanisms. In response, females have developed internal mechanisms to weed out inferior genetic contributors. Under the influence of differing parental investment theory, women are at a higher risk of wasting time and provisions on genetically inferior offspring; therefore, reproductive systems have been selected for that allow women to retain the best sperm from the best male specimen.[101]

On the male side of things, chemicals in semen have been selected for that have an antidepressant effect on women. This may have the effect of making women unconsciously seek mating with men to positively affect their psychological states.[102] Other weapons men use in their semen are follicle stimulating hormone (FSH) and luteinizing hormone (LH). These hormones may work to help men stimulate ovulation in their sex partners.[103] Another mechanism men have developed to make sure their sperm are the victors in sperm competition within the female's vaginas are seminal compounds that block competitors' sperm from getting to the woman's egg. Also, men's semen comes with immunosuppressive compounds that lower female immune defenses to protect their sperm from being attacked.

But, of course, on the woman's side of things, she has immunological agents that are set up to attack unrecognized intruders. That is why men who are in committed romances with women are often more successful in impregnating them.[104]

Dr. Gorelik also describes sexual manipulation by men and women through psychological means as part of sexual conflict: facial expressions, verbal and nonverbal communication, the emulation of the behavior of the other person (mirroring), and other subtle means. These subconscious events can indirectly influence the brain chemistry of the opposite sex.[105]

Again, at the root of these elements of sexual conflict are sex differences developed over long periods of selection time. To illustrate some of these psychological sex differences, let's look to Dr. Irina Trofimova's article, "Do Psychological Sex Differences Reflect Evolutionary Bisexual Partitioning?" which gives us an excellent list to start. See if they ring true with your experience:

Consistent Sex Differences in Psychological Abilities
- Males tend to have higher rates of risk and sensation seeking, criminal behavior, and openness to experience and to mating with strangers than females (Costa et al., 2001)[106]
- Males are three and a half times more likely to die from all accidental causes and two and a half times more likely to die in road accidents than are females (Kruger, 2004)[107]
- Males have higher rates of impulsivity and poor compliance with routine and prescribed behavior (Struber, et al., 2008; Cross et al., 2011) [108][109]
- Men use aggressive behavior more often than women. Recent reports suggest that men use more physical aggression, whereas women use more verbal aggression (Archer, 2004; Idaho State Department of Education, 2013), [110][111]
- Males have greater upper body strength and physical endurance and faster tempo than females, especially youths (Bishop, et al., 1987)[112]
- Males have superiority in mechanical reasoning, spatial abilities, and ability to simplify and generalize new information. This coincides with a tendency of males to perceive ambivalent objects as more simple, easy to handle, and not challenging (Halpern, 2012)[113]

- Females have higher fluency with words and better verbal memory, verbal analogy, spelling, language-related reasoning, and naming objects (Halpern, 2012)[114]
- Females exhibit significantly higher empathic, teaching, parenting, rule-driven, and imitative behavior, and males exhibit significantly higher exploratory and competitive behavior from a very early age. This is consistent with their choice of toys and later choice of profession (Baron-Cohen, 2003, 2011)[115]
- Females exhibit better communication skills and use of language; they interrupt less and show more tentative speech than males (Leaper & Robnett, 2011)[116]
- Females have higher rates of social endurance, extroversion, and agreeableness (Trofimova, 2010)[117]
- In jobs with a need for single ability, either verbal or physical, there is a preponderance of females in social and secretarial services and in children's education (more than 90 percent of US bank tellers, receptionists, registered nurses, and preschool and kindergarten teachers are women) and a preponderance of males in physically demanding jobs (more than 90 percent of firefighters, mechanics, and pest exterminators are men) (Browne, 2002)[118]
- Women are more sensitive to punishment (Cross et al., 2011)[119]
- Cross-culturally, females are superior to males at recognizing emotions in faces, voice, gestures, and nonverbal cues and at interpreting a range of mental states (Baron-Cohen, 2011)[120]
- Females are superior to males at perception, discrimination, and remembering taste odors, auditory tones, and colors (Halpern, 2012)[121]

Well, what do you think?

Remember, these psychological traits represent averages across populations in Western societies. Therefore, there will be exceptions. Even so, does your life experience agree with these sex differences regarding many of the people you know? In "It's Funny Because it is True (Because it Evokes our Evolved Psychology)," Dr. Barry X Kuhle reveals why the comedy of Chris Rock makes people laugh. He points out that they find it humorous because it rings true with what most people recognize as human sexual nature.[122]

Master Manipulators

Psychological phenomena such as thoughts, emotions, and behaviors are a reflection of sex differences at the molecular and anatomical levels. As a result, male psychology was formed by selection to be interested in a variety of sex partners and to presume that a woman is receptive to sex, whether or not that is actually the case.[123] Three other psychological adaptations to sexual conflict that Dr. Gorelik lists are mate-guarding[124] and sexual and emotional jealousy.[125] However, when there is sexual cooperation in play, reciprocity, status, and protection are employed by the male. In these ways, men may employ nurturing and positive treatment to guard their mates against cheating.[126] Both types of sexual conflict, at the molecular level and the psychological level, revolve around manipulation, counter-manipulation, and defense against manipulation.

Dr. David Buss, in *The Evolution of Desire*, also outlines sexual conflict very effectively. He broadly defines it as one sex interfering with the goals and desires of the other. He starts by giving one of the most common examples of how a man circumvents a sexual goal of many women, who want greater emotional commitment and higher resource investment, when he seeks sex without much investment.

On the other hand, women who call for extended courtship and heavy investment interfere with many men's short-term mating strategy.

The experience of sexual conflict triggers emotions that we have inherited from our ancestors that prompt us to psychologically do something about it. Psychological reactions include anger, distress, and upset, and they help motivate actions that remedy the situation and prevent it from happening again in the future.

Near and Far Sighted

One of the most common areas of sexual conflict between men and women concerns sexual access or availability. Men have a tendency to seek sex while only minimally investing in their partner. They try to protect their resources. Women have long term-sexual strategies and they look for signs of investment by the male. Another common area of conflict is over-perceived sex appeal. When a person is ignored by someone they seek, there is often resentment on the part of the shunned. There can be a lot of anger attached to not being "good enough" for the desired date. An additional area of sexual conflict that is very important and displays another sex difference is men's tendency to over-perceive a woman's sexual interest. This male over-perception bias causes some men to become sexually pushy and can lead to sexual aggression in spite of a woman's reluctance.

> Sexual aggression can be classified as forced sexual intimacy, sex without getting mutual agreement, and unauthorized sexual touching.

This scenario is at the heart of much of the sexual conflict on today's college campuses in Western society. What adds insult to injury in this regrettable situation is that women understandably react very negatively to these violations. In one study, women were asked to rate 147 potentially upsetting actions that men could take against them. These women rated sexual aggression very near the possible maximum. No other kinds of offensive acts, like verbal and physical abuse, even came close to being perceived and received as negatively as sexual aggression.

To make matters worse, men are much less bothered by women who are sexually aggressive. As a matter of fact, the same study showed that on average men are *less than half* as upset as women about sexual aggression from the opposite sex. Some men said they would even find it arousing if women were sexually aggressive towards them. This represents a very important disconnect between the lens that men see sexual activity through versus the lens women see it through. Men incessantly underestimate how unacceptable women find sexual aggression. In the same way, a logically consistent finding is that women consistently overestimate how upsetting sexual aggression by a woman towards a man is considered. They overestimate as much as men underestimate sexual aggression's negative impact on women.[127] Men expect women to see things sexually the way they do, and women expect men to see things sexually the way they do. Understanding this situation is crucial to addressing the problems brought about by sexual aggression throughout Western society.

Dr. Buss sums up the situation this way: "Acquiring knowledge about gender differences in perceptions of sexual aggression might be one step toward reducing sexual conflict."[128]

That is one of the most important goals of *Battles of the Sexes*.

A Need for Education

The vast majority of young men and women in Western societies have no education about these sex differences, especially in the area of sexual aggression.

One of my first inklings of the lack of education in this area happened many years ago when the fitness center at our university was remodeled. There were young women in my personal conditioning class that I had seen working out in the cardiovascular conditioning room, which was on the second floor of the facility. Before the remodeling project began, I saw them often, and always encouraged them and applauded their efforts. After the remodeling project started, the entrance to the building changed. When you checked in, you had to walk by the weight lifting area that was located on the first floor behind glass walls. I noticed I hadn't seen the young women from my class for a while, so I asked where they had been and why they stopped coming. I was expecting them to say that they were too busy with their social life or homework, but their answers surprised me.

They said they had stopped coming because the entrance had been changed. They now had to walk by the glass walls of the weight training area to get to the stairs of the cardio room. They didn't like the guys in the weight room staring at them, which always happened, so they decided it wasn't worth coming until they changed the entrance back.

I said to them, "I thought you ladies liked guys staring at you."

They said, "Not in that way and in that place."

They perceived the stares as a form of sexual aggression and it was off-putting to them. After learning more about the research in this area, it started to make sense.

Women Only

This female sex difference may be a big part of the reason why the Women's Personal Conditioning class was so successful. At the height of the program, Women's Personal Conditioning was being chosen by around two thirds of the female students who were taking classroom-based personal conditioning. I realize now that many statements from my dissertation research[129] had a direct connection to this regrettable situation of sexual conflict. When asked why they chose a female-specific P.E. class, some of the focus group's answers from my dissertation reflected sexual conflict rationales.

"I wasn't looking forward to having guys look at me at the gym, but this class was helpful to get over that."

"It is normally stressful to go to the gym. I don't like to go to the gym."

"In this class, we got to focus on women and there is no pressure to be 'on' for the sexual tension that there is when guys are involved."

"With all women, there isn't a lot of competition. It makes you feel stronger. It is intimidating with men around. It makes you self-conscious. It's more comfortable around just women."

"I liked it because I didn't feel like I had to look cute; I wasn't trying to impress anybody. If I woke up in the morning and didn't feel like putting my makeup on, I didn't have to, and nobody was judging me for it."[130]

The focus groups were conducted on the last day of each class. I took note at the time that when it comes to a fitness venue, many college females prefer that it be business oriented. What they don't want is a physical activity environment where courting is one of the goals and where they may feel awkward unless they are prepared to be "on." I now realize that some of this compartmentalizing desire may stem from the collegiate environment these young women experience.

Hookup Culture

Without going into too much detail here because we will examine it carefully in relationship to college women in chapter ten, let's say that a more impersonal and sometimes combative relational environment, especially for women, has emerged on college campuses in the last decade.

It is called **hookup culture**.

Basically, it calls for young men and women to have varying degrees of sexual relations with people they have perhaps just met, sometimes as casually as at a dance. In other words, it consists of sexual relations without accompanying emotional relationships. This casual attitude toward sexual relationships and disregard for romance has been clearly shown in previous chapters to go against the heart of classic female mating strategies. It has to have had a chilling and intimidating effect on interpersonal relationships between college women and men.

That college men would be in favor of a hookup culture is not surprising. It is *very* surprising, however, that college women would go along with it.

He Always Ignores My Feelings

One of the other key areas of sexual conflict concerns the reluctance of men to share their feelings openly. David Buss writes that among newlywed couples 45 percent of women in comparison to only 24 percent of men complain that their spouses fail to share their true feelings. While dating, 25 percent of women complain that men ignore their feelings and it increases to 30 percent by the first year of marriage. By the fourth year of marriage, 59 percent of women say their husbands ignore their feelings. Only about half that percentage of men share this sentiment, with 12 percent complaining the first year of marriage and only 32 percent complaining by the fourth year.

As you should expect by this point, there is a sex difference in the value placed on emotional intimacy in a relationship.

Escalated Sexual Conflict

After learning about the impersonal environment young women live in during college, their desire for an all-women physical activity venue becomes more understandable. They are coming to class from a college social life that contains many types of sexual conflict and they just want a place where they can rest from it, relax, and take care of their wellness among same-sex friends.

Unfortunately, hooking up and its related miscommunication isn't the worst form of sexual conflict on campus.

As inferred in the hookup scenario, sexual harassment may be an outgrowth of the environment and biology on college campuses, as well as workplaces. Sexual harassment doesn't happen randomly. Studies have shown that more women than men report having been sexually harassed (it should also be remembered that on average women feel more distress when experiencing sexual aggression than do men).[131] There is also the factor of what types of women are most likely harassed. They are usually young, single women. Women above the age of 45 are less likely to be harassed, revealing the connection to male sexuality as men gravitate towards women with higher reproductive potential.[132]

Reactions to sexual harassment may have biological roots. When women were asked how they would feel if a coworker asked them to have sex, 63 percent said they would take it as an insult and 17 percent said they would be flattered.[133] Men's attitudes were the polar opposite. Only 15 percent of men were insulted, while 67 percent said they would be flattered. Clearly, when it comes to casual sex in the workplace, men and women once again see through vastly different lenses.

The final forms of escalated sexual conflict we will look at are sexual assault and rape. One of the great misconceptions about rape is that it usually happens as a result of a stranger jumping out from behind some bushes. One study showed that 15 percent of college women had been subjected to undesired sexual intercourse during a date[134]—*with someone they knew*. Nearly all rapists are males, and most victims are females. Most rapists come from low socioeconomic groups. The average ages of women that are raped are similar to those of the ones who suffer sexual harassment. In one study of over 10,000 rape victims, females age 16-35 were more likely to be raped than any other age category. In fact, 85 percent of all rape victims are younger than 36 years old.[135]

One of the most sobering findings about men's greater tendency to rape comes from a study in which they were asked to envision a hypothetical situation. In this imaginary scenario, they were asked if they had the opportunity to force sex on a woman with no chance of being caught, no chance of anyone else knowing, no risk of STIs, and no risk to their reputations, would they take it? *Around 35 percent said there was some likelihood they would assault the woman.*[136]

Another study showed that 27 percent of men might also force sex on a woman under those conditions.[137] This means that around one third of men, according to these studies, have potential to rape. The good news is that around two thirds of men are *not* potential rapists. Nonetheless, that one third figure is a distressing statistic.

At this point we should again mention that we wrote *Battles of the Sexes* in consultation with the Sexual Assault Center of Nashville, who supplied us with many helpful facts and insights on sexual assault and rape, such as:

- 1 out of every 6 American women have been the victim of either attempted or completed rape, which means numerically that 17.7 million American women have been the victims of attempted or completed rape.

- About 3 percent of American men, or 2.78 million, have been the victims of attempted or completed rape.
- About 25 percent of American college females have reported being the survivors of rape or attempted rape.
- More than 50 percent of all sexual assault and rape is reported to have happened within one mile of the victim's home or at their place of residence.
- Finally, sexual assault is one of the crimes that goes most unreported at a rate of 54 percent not being reported.[138]

An object lesson in all of this occurred in Nashville in 2013 at Vanderbilt University. In what has become known as the Vanderbilt Rape Case, a female student was allegedly raped while incapacitated by drugs and unconscious in a dorm room on campus. Four former Vanderbilt football players were accused of the crime. At the time of this writing, three have been convicted. Of the three, one is serving a seventeen-year sentence and the other two are each serving fifteen years. It should be understood that because these are aggravated rape sentences, the convicted young men must serve them out fully without any possibility of parole. This means they will not be free until they are in their late 30s.

Obviously, this was a very traumatic, hurtful event in the female victim's life. Her life may never be the same. The young men's lives will rightfully never be the same either as after they are released and for the remainder of their days, they will be registered sex offenders. Sexual assault and rape are very serious crimes and are obviously a ruinous activity for everyone involved. As the attorneys in the case said, there are no winners.[139] The only way to win is to avoid being involved in any way in nonconsensual sex. Obtaining clear consent is of paramount importance!

(In case no one has drilled that into your head already. Because it's important.)

Other related studies have shown that sexually coercive men display a certain set of distinct traits. They tend to be women-haters, believe that women eagerly desire to be raped, are impulsive, hostile, not very agreeable, have little empathy, are hyper-masculine, and are very promiscuous.[139]

With all of this information about sexual conflict as a backdrop, it's easy to see why the young women in the Women's Personal Conditioning class may have had some of the feelings they did about males. It also can help us better understand why some college women would seek an environment where sexual conflict was minimized. To see if feelings towards the class and its effects lasted over time, I conducted thirty-two in-depth interviews with former class members up to twenty-six months after they had finished the course. This is what some of them shared:

*"I love the bonding time with other friends, sorority sisters, and new faces. It also helps when classes are gender-specific because women usually don't want to work around men, as it can be intimidating or off-putting altogether. So now that I am not in the class, I usually exercise with other female friends, by myself, or with my dog. The only man I ever care to be around when I'm working out is my husband." - **Michelle, 2012***

"I really enjoyed that the class was only for women because personally, working out with guys can be a little intimidating. Men and women have completely different ways of working out and I think that women appreciate

having a class that is geared toward their bodies and personal health." - **Simone, 2012**

"An all-women's class I think is important because we may feel intimidated by a male in the room during a workout. We're not letting on how we feel out loud because we may get embarrassed or we may think they will judge us in a way we don't like unless they understand us. All women have a common feeling when it comes to looks or how we feel, so I think it's easier to talk openly about that when it is an all-women's class."
- **Terry, 2014**

"I love the all-women aspect of the class. It gave us a sense of closeness—our bond being stronger. In WPC, there was no pressure to impress the opposite sex, and that helped us stay focused on the reason we enrolled in the class." - **Jordan, 2012**[140]

Sexual conflicts in a fitness arena can arise from one sex's optimal fitness strategies differing from the others. One comment from a young man who was in a co-ed personal conditioning class reflects the contrasting point of view of males in this situation. His comment was part of a pilot study to get young men's perspectives on mixed gender P.E. classes.[141]

"I think it [standard coed personal conditioning] has a positive impact on my experience. Seeing hot girls working out while I work out was enjoyable."[142]

R-E-S-P-E-C-T

You can see that the potential for heartache and heartbreak is high in this world of sexual conflict. This is particularly true when the underlying causes lie largely outside the conscious understanding of women and men who are involved in the conflict. Dr. Gregory Gorelik describes it like this: "In case of culture, individual level sexual conflict is evident at the level of social structures, institutions, practices, and beliefs. Thus, gender politics may be a different level of analysis for the same phenomena that can be understood from other theoretical perspectives."[143]

In other words, sexual conflict, much of which is caused by clashing biological conflicts of interest, may annoyingly be the root cause of many of our societal and political conflicts (Barney from *How I Met Your Mother* may have been on to something). What makes this deplorable situation even worse is that one of the greatest causes for this sexual conflict is a lack of awareness of it's biological roots. After our explanation of the biology of human sexual conflict, you are much better prepared to *actually do something* about it. We believe that, as Sir Francis Bacon said, "knowledge is power." You now have the power to empower a new concept: sexual empathy for yourselves, and even more importantly, for those you love.

———————— A SARAH SUMMARY: ————————

- The battle of the sexes is, in essence, the lack of accountability for the needs of the opposite sex due to the conflicting natural mating strategies developed over time. Women generally seek long term emotional commitment and resource investment, while men may be hard wired to "hit it and quit it," which

is why college hookup culture is heavily skewed toward the preference of one gender to the detriment of the other.
- Men have a higher propensity to force sexual acts on women. It is important for men and women to understand this phenomenon to potentially prevent this from occurring by bringing it out of the unconscious mind to the conscious.

Chapter 9

. . . .

Resolving Sexual Conflict Through Sexual Empathy, Sexual Respect, and Sexual Synergy

"Be kind, for everyone you meet is fighting a hard battle."
PLATO

Sexual Empathy

The more I have experienced life, the more I have learned the truth of Plato's famous quote. You never know what people are going through, but in almost all cases, it's a safe bet that even if they aren't fighting a hard battle right now, they have at some point. This kind of attitude and disposition is the heart of empathy. If someone really wants to raise their level of empathy, they must get to know the other person better—get to know their perspective and outlook on life. An excellent way to accomplish this is to carefully observe their lived experience. As Harper Lee wisely wrote in *To Kill a Mockingbird*:

> "You never really understand a person until you consider things from their point of view—until you climb into their skin and walk around in it."

I didn't have that kind of experience until I was conducting my dissertation research. Then, I took a gender-specific look at the day-to-day experience of young women in college P.E. classes and came away a changed person. I realized how much I hadn't known about their way of seeing things. But I was willing to learn. As a matter of fact, I received what I consider one of the greatest compliments of my entire career from a Women's Personal Conditioning student during the dissertation interviews.

> *"I definitely felt like I had a positive relationship with Coach Malone. Coach was always smiles. We talked about hormones... I couldn't imagine talking about hormones and how women react to things, but with Coach, it was easy. He wasn't uncomfortable. It was blunt, and he could relate it to his wife or family. He always ended up seeming like one of the girls. Not as in a girlfriend, but he'd talk like any female coach would, with as much compassion and care in his voice."[144]*

My years of teaching the Women's Personal Conditioning class gave me a new kind of empathy: **sexual empathy**. Recently, I defined sexual empathy on Urban Dictionary.

Sexual empathy: The ability to understand and respect the perspective of the opposite sex.

One of our major goals is to raise the SEX IQ of our readers in order to empower sexual empathy in them. To us, sexual empathy is one of the most important types of empathy that exists. This empathy can lead to **sexual synergy**—the kind of synergy human females and males have employed for millions of years.

Barbara Annis and Keith Merron have a similar belief in *Gender Intelligence*. They believe that while it's crucial to comprehend that men and women often communicate, address problems, form decisions, handle emotions, and handle stress differently, the realization shouldn't stop there. We need to understand that the differences have purpose, deep meaning, and *value*. The paramount reason that our species has been so successful for millions of years is directly due to sex differences. These differences are designed for cooperation and being complementary to the opposite sex, not for competition.

The differences that began in our hunting and gathering years are still apparent on college campuses and even in corporations.[145] Dr. Helen Fisher in *The First Sex* describes women as predominantly thinking holistically and contextually. She says that women have a tendency to arrange their thinking in webs of factors. They tend to see more relationships between different factors and many more potential possibilities before making decisions. Men, on the other hand, have a tendency to focus on a certain issue, block out extraneous data, and move in a regimented fashion towards the goal.[146] Annis and Merron find the difference in the two ways of thinking positively exciting. Not because of how far apart they are, but by the potential possibilities when they're combined!

Puzzle Pieces

Instead of thinking one way or the other, what would happen if they were combined? What would happen if we could combine those strengths, those two perfectly good ways of thinking, when we make important decisions?

Dr. Fisher says men and women are made to put their heads together, both professionally and personally. As the sexes join together to understand their individual strengths, they both have an opportunity to gain crucial insight into the other's world. Both have the chance to accomplish new empathy and rapport. When women and men are able to understand the nature of their gender differences, assumptions and misunderstandings are reduced and their relationship clarity increases. They have increased appreciation for each other's behavior, and actually get profound insight into their own behavior as well.[147] We agree wholeheartedly and applaud the intelligence and sensitivity it takes to come to this enlightened conclusion. This is the kind of thinking and insight we need more of throughout Western societies.

Focus on the Positive

Dr. Paul Zak, once again, also gets to the heart of the advantages of the differences between females and males. He talks about some of the advantages of having high testosterone—things like increased ability for athletic performance because of the increased muscle mass and bone density. High testosterone also comes in handy if you need to run into a burning building to rescue survivors or attack a fortified enemy position. He summarizes by saying it is especially useful any time we face a situation that calls for risk taking, raw courage, strength, and bodily speed. He also points out that a male strength is an increased willingness to punish wrongdoers. An example he gives is the person at the beach that has the music turned up disturbingly loud—it is usually a male who will confront him. We have discussed the downside of testosterone and will continue to do so, but for a moment, let's realize that these characteristics are no small thing and aren't always negative. Remember the earlier example of his that we cited; when it comes to the successful functioning of Western society, he points out with the famous Donner expedition the need for a fine and complementary balance of men and women working together. Over millions of years of natural and sexual selection, a two-pronged approach to species survival has come about. Either gender is capable of violence, competition, and aggression, along with compassion and bonding. But, men being hormonally predisposed with higher testosterone levels makes them take the lead on aggressive tendencies, while the higher levels of oxytocin and estrogen predispose women to take the lead in compassion. As a result, the men in the Donner party leading the wagon train west chose to take an aggressive shortcut to reach California quicker. Survivor accounts reveal that the women of the Donner party were dead set against taking the risk of the unproven route.

I wonder if they said, "I told you so."

Dr. Zak concludes that the predominantly male route of aggressiveness and risk-taking can absolutely get you killed. On the other hand, too little risk-taking could have meant that most pioneers, not just the Donner party, might have stayed home and worked for wages in Boston, New York, or some other Eastern city, and never would have gotten their piece of California or Montana to become self-sufficient farmers.[148]

David Buss also has many good things to add in this area. He points out that we are not slaves to the sex roles that have originated in natural and sexual selection. Knowledge of our differing desires and the benefits and costs of different strategies allows us to choose from a varied mating menu. Understanding why sexual strategies have developed and the adaptive problems they were designed to address gives us a powerful tool to change behavior. The essence of this tool is the ability to develop sexual empathy. Once we can appreciate the problems and challenges both sexes are facing, largely because of the mismatch between inherited sexual nature and rapidly changing culture, we can begin to feel empathy and understanding for both sexes.

Women *and* men, as Dr. Buss rightly points out, have faced many of the same adaptive pressures over time and share many common psychological solutions. For example, both sexes place a very high value on reciprocal love, intelligence, and dependability in a lifelong mate. Both seek lifelong mates who are loyal, worthy of trust, and generally cooperative. Both sexes also look for life partners who will not incur catastrophic losses. The two sexes also have many common biological functions (i.e. sweating, digestion, etc.). Recognition of this common biology and psychology is an important step towards sexual cooperation.

Equally Important, But Not the Same

What also must be acknowledged are sex differences brought about by *differing* adaptive challenges faced by men and women over the millions of years of human history. Because women have always shouldered the responsibility for nourishing their infants, women have breasts that can provide milk. Because natural fertilization occurs internally in women, ancestral men have always been uncertain of their fatherhood. As a result, they have developed a mate preference for women who will be sexually loyal and empower their paternity certainty and have also developed strong sexual jealousy.

Sexual selection pressures have made men more inclined to choose youth and physical attractiveness and made women look for status, maturity, professional success, the ability to protect, and abundant economic resources in men. Relatedly, of course, men are much more interested in casual sex without emotional commitment, sexual variety, and sexual fantasy. Dr. Buss uses social media as a demonstration of these differences. Tinder, he says, has many more men than women that are looking for casual sex. Ashley Madison is used mostly by married men seeking variety. SeekingArrangement.com mostly matches men with high social status and economic resources with beautiful young women who want to connect with them.

Understanding the biological forces behind these kinds of behaviors and strategies is the first step towards sexual empathy.

As Dr. Buss writes, we are empowered now, more than ever, to shape our collective future. *Just because deception, abuse, and sexual coercion may emanate from our selected mating strategies doesn't mean that they are justified.* This is where we can use our frontal cortex to override immoral behavior. Sexual empathy can, and should, be at its highest level among humans.

Like Peanut Butter and Jelly

Women and men working together can become more than the sum of their parts. Shared human mating resources oftentimes go well beyond reproductively-related essentials to include protection from dangers, mutual fighting of enemies, mutual friendship networks, the education of children, loyalty through good times and bad, and nurturing of each other when there are life setbacks. Each of these couple characteristics helps define our overall human nature. A profound respect of the other sex should come from the realization that we have always depended on each other for the complementary skills and resources that were required for survival and reproduction. Also, we have historically depended on the other sex for the fulfillment of our desires. This scenario may be responsible for the unique feeling of completeness that humans experience when they fall into the warm embrace of lasting, romantic love. Dr. Buss concludes that a lifetime alliance of love is a triumphant achievement of human mating strategies.[149]

We couldn't agree more.

That is sexual empathy and sexual synergy at their best. This special female and male sexual synergy relationship has been the secret of our success and yes, even our survival, for at least the last two million years. We don't see that changing anytime soon!

─────────── A SARAH SUMMARY: ───────────

- Sexual empathy involves understanding and respecting the perspective of the opposite sex to ensure cooperation instead of competition.
- It is important to put focus on the positive aspects and contributions that come from each gender's unique biological makeup.
- The genders are equal, but to act like they are exactly the same is foolishness.

PART IV

College Days All the Way
to Marriage Ways

Chapter 10

. . . .

Romance Wreckers—An Ounce of Prevention for Her

"We are what we repeatedly do.
Excellence, then is not an act but a habit"
Aristotle

"Knowledge without execution is useless."
Tony Robbins

The Overwhelm of Femininity

I am writing this part specifically for college women. I know that you are going through one of the most exciting, tumultuous, and challenging times of your lives. You're expected to hold down a job, take care of your academics, and keep up with your social lives, all while looking fit, healthy, and otherwise attractive.

And this didn't start when you got to college.

137

You probably have been living under this pressure since the middle of your high school years at least. This increasing pressure has led to higher levels of depression (over 20 percent), increased suicide attempts, more self-mutilation, and increased eating disorders amongst women.[150] For college women, in my personal experience, this seems to have led to lowered self-esteem. In fact, one study showed that during college, self-esteem for males rises as it falls for females.[151] In talking with a longtime sorority adviser, I learned this can lead to an acceptance of bad relationships by women and irresponsible use of alcohol. Finally, it can lead to something we spoke of earlier: a general lack of exercise combined with increased addiction to junk foods.

On a national scale, 89 percent of female college students revealed that they felt overwhelmed by their task load, which is 15 percent more than males. Around 98 percent of college women said that they felt hopeless in the previous year, 9 percent higher than males. Approximately 57 percent of female college students reported high anxiety, 17 percent higher than males. Around 89 percent of college women felt exhausted, but not from exercise, which was 14 percent higher than college men.[152]

Again, this situation didn't start in college for these women. High school females are twice as likely to say that they felt overwhelmed by all they had to accomplish. First-year female college students were 13 percent less likely than men to report high levels of emotional health.[153]

Swipe Left, Swipe Right

To add to all of these challenging situations, the relationship arena in college for most students has become much more impersonal and less romantic with the emergence of the hookup culture. It's been described as an unprecedented time in the history of sexual relations.[154]

In the US, the age at which young adults first marry and have children has been delayed dramatically. At the same time, puberty is being entered at younger and younger ages. This has created a situation where young people are able to physiologically reproduce, but are not psychologically or socially ready to create permanent bonds and their own independent family unit.[155] It has been suggested by some research that these developmental shifts may be behind the increase in sexual hookups of young adults throughout Western societies. Experts in this area are asserting that hookups are becoming more and more ingrained in our popular culture due to sexually selective preferences combined with an accommodating social and sexual culture. Hookups are described as running the gamut of sexual behaviors, from kissing and oral sex to penetrative intercourse, but the thing that is different in hookup culture is that these acts often are done without any promise of, or desire expressed for, a more traditional, romantic love relationship.[156] In other words, sexual behavior outside of traditional, committed, romantic relationships has become more and more socially acceptable in the twenty-first century.

The media has acted as a major inaccurate source of sex education with a sensationalized portrayal of sexuality.[158] The underlying message of magazines, movies, search engines, TV shows, and the lyrics of music work together to create a permissive sexual ambiance. The media paint the picture of uncommitted sex as being both physically and emotionally pleasurable without any strings attached. Movies such as 2009's *Hooking Up* and 2011's *No Strings Attached* are good examples of this very additude.

Where is the Love?

Is this hookup culture really realistic in light of what we know about sex differences, specifically in regard to male preferences for variety and females being the choosier sex?

In one study of the morning after a hookup, 82 percent of men and 57 percent of women said they were mostly glad they had done it. That margin of difference between male and female reaction is significant.[159]

In another study of 832 college students, only 26 percent of women, but a full 50 percent of men, reported feeling positive after a hookup, while 49 percent of women and 26 percent of men had a negative reaction.[160] In another qualitative study of 187 students, 35 percent felt regretful, 27 percent good, 20 percent satisfied, 11 percent confused, 9 percent proud, 7 percent excited or nervous, 5 percent uncomfortable, and 2 percent desirable or wanted.[161] When you add up all of the negative reactions, you get 44 percent. That seems substantial for an act that is advertised as pleasurable and care-free by the media. Another interesting insight was applied by this same study. It seems that during the hookup, 65 percent of the participants felt good, aroused, or excited, 17 percent desirable or wanted, 17 percent nothing in particular, or were focused on the hookup, 8 percent embarrassed or regretful, 7 percent nervous or scared, 6 percent confused, and 5 percent proud.[162] It seems that in the heat of the moment, priorities can change.[163] An interesting study by that very name showcased how this works for young men, and it's very important that young women know about it.

Thinking with the Wrong Head

Dr. Dan Ariely and Dr. George Lowenstein of MIT took a look at how sexual arousal impacts college men's judgement and moral backbone. They asked college men to answer questions about their moral boundaries while in two different mental states: unaroused or aroused (by masturbating to pornography). In the aroused state, these young men were about twice as likely to consider tying up a sex partner, envision being attracted to a 12-year-old girl, tell a young woman that they loved her when they didn't to get her to have sex, keep trying to have sex with a woman even after she said no, give women alcohol or drugs to increase the chances for sex, and even entertain the thought of sex with animals.

Clearly, these men lost their sense of empathy and respect for women as their arousal increased. Men have a tendency to underestimate the impact of arousal on their judgement.

Don't you make that mistake.

According to Ariely and Lowenstein, the best way for men to practice self-control is to avoid those situations while they are still in an unaroused state (and can think clearly). To avoid the possibility of date rape or hookup rape, they suggest women also become aware of this phenomenon and, even though it is no justification, realize that sexual arousal strongly and adversely affects men's ability to do the right thing and makes them more vulnerable to displaying sexually aggressive behavior.[164] I wonder how many 'heat of the moment' sexual coercion scenarios this accounts for. No matter how you look at this, everyone loses. Regrettably, situations like this may contribute to the number of young women and men who have negative feelings after casual sex.

The Regret of Hit-It-and-Quit-It

In another study of 1,468 college students on sexual activity, 27 percent felt embarrassed, 25 percent reported emotional difficulties, 21 percent felt loss of respect, and 10 percent experienced difficulties with a steady partner.[165] A Canadian study of 270 college-aged students revealed that 72 percent regretted at least one incidence of sexual activity in the past.[166] In a study of 152 college women, 74 percent had either few or some regrets after a hookup; 61 percent had few regrets, 23 percent had no regrets, 13 percent had some regrets, and 3 percent had many regrets.[167]

In a related study, college women's, but not college men's, depression symptoms increased as their number of sexual partners in a year increased.[168] Dr. Garcia and Dr. Reiber wrote that the differences between a person's desires and behaviors, particularly in respect to sociosexual relationships, can have dramatic effects on physical and mental health. Despite the allure of hookups, research shows that people, especially young women, take part in these behaviors even when they feel uncomfortable doing so.[169] They also have a tendency to overestimate others' comfort with hookups.

Misperception of sexual norms is a potential driver for people, *especially young women,* to behave in ways they do not personally believe in.

This is a very important point. The authors found that 78 percent of college students overestimated others' comfort with hookup behaviors, with men especially overestimating women's comfort with the hookups.[170]

Walk of Guilt

Part of the reason for this over perception by men is that they may feel less guilt than women over hooking up. In a study of 169 sexually experienced women and men in single's bars, only 32 percent of men said they would feel guilty about having intercourse with someone they just met compared to 72 percent of women.[171] The percentage of women feeling guilty was over twice that of men. Other research shows that women have a tendency to seek more emotional involvement in sexual encounters than men.

A hint as to what is behind these sex differences when it comes to worry: In a study of 507 college students, more women than men hoped a relationship would be the result of a hookup. Just 4 percent of men and 8 percent of women outright expected a traditional romantic relationship to be an outcome. But 29 percent of men and 43 percent of women idealistically hoped for such an outcome.[172]

Dr. Garcia and Dr. Reiber state it is likely that a substantial portion of young adults today feel compelled to publicly take part in hookups, while actually desiring both expedited sexual gratification and more stable romantic attachments.[173] To make things even more complicated, there is the ever-present issue of the prevalence and use of alcohol and other drugs. In a study of 118 freshmen female college students, participants shared that in 64 percent of cases hookups followed alcohol use. The average number of drinks in these encounters was three.[174] When you look at this college hookup scene as a whole, it presents a pretty negative picture.

Most alarming of all is the relationship of hookup culture with nonconsensual sex. In a study of 178 college men and women, the participants revealed that most of their experience with unwanted sex occurred while engaged in a hookup. Regarding unwanted sex, **78 percent took place during a hookup**, 14 percent during an ongoing relationship, and 8 percent on a date.[175]

This is a monumentally important insight!

There are, and have been, many large-scale efforts taking place on college campuses across Western societies to decrease the amount of sexual coercion, sexual assault, and rape. The research insight that most nonconsensual sex occurs in the context of hookup culture sheds new light on what needs to be done to decrease the incidences of all kinds of sexual aggression.

Alcohol Made Me Do It

Additionally, Dr Donna Freitas, who has studied hookup culture extensively, says that 41 percent of the students in her survey reported

144 | *Battles of the Sexes*

being *profoundly* upset about hooking up. Some of them even likened the experience to abuse. She outlines the case that alcohol, hooking up, and sexual assault are often related. Dr. Freitas quotes a study that reveals that 26 percent of students who were freshmen or sophomores had sex with someone they had just met while they were under the influence of alcohol. Around 40 percent of these freshmen or sophomore students had sex with someone they knew but were not in a relationship with while drinking alcohol. Within that same study, 44 percent of women reported at least one unwanted sexual episode while in college and, **again, 90 percent of these unwanted sexual encounters happened during a hookup.** Of the total reported incidents of nonconsensual sex, 76 percent involved alcohol. Having alcohol in the mix blurred whether consent had been given. The researchers discovered that often the victim was too drunk to properly give consent and didn't remember what happened the next day.

Several of the women Dr. Freitas interviewed said it never occurred to their partner to ask for, or wait for, consent. Talking is not what the hookup was about—getting it done is usually the object. In hookup culture on campus, students are conditioned to think that sex just happens, especially when you're drunk. The goal is then not to cry about it the next day since that creates drama, which defeats the purpose of the hookup. Dr. Freitas applauded the 2011 Obama administration letter pressuring college administrators to better uphold policies regarding sexual assault, but she makes an excellent point when she says that her optimism about it is tempered by her worry that the vast majority of colleges will fail to address hookup culture's very intimate relationship to rape culture (as it is called on many campuses). In her experience, many colleges have either barely acknowledged hookup culture, have avoided conversation about it because of potential scandal or because it couldn't be a problem on *their* campus, or because they don't regard it as a problem, period.

Sign the Consent Form

Most sexual assault programming Dr. Freitas has encountered still centers on language, for instance that no means no and yes means yes, showcasing the importance of gaining consent. While this type of education is of course important, in many ways it has become basically useless in light of hookup culture.

Hooking up is an activity where communication itself is seen as counterproductive to success. Therefore, solely focusing on teaching the practice of gaining consent is insufficient in the often drunk and silent hookup culture. Dr. Freitas contends, and we agree, that hookup culture and sexual assault must be *addressed together* if we want to end sexual assault. Sexual assault must be challenged in the light of a widespread student culture that teaches students that yes and no are unimportant, that apathy about sexual intimacy is the desired norm, and that whatever happens under the influence of alcohol is justifiable and unavoidable.[176]

Obviously, we have to look at hookup culture as being a huge and integral part of the problem, even though it is often not widely recognized as such (if it's recognized at all).

In *Mating Intelligence Unleashed,* Dr. Glenn Geher and Dr. Scott Barry Kaufman describe the hookup culture that has been the norm for more than a decade on college campuses. They cite statistics showing that 65-80 percent of undergraduate college students have hooked up at least once during their time in college.

What is causing this increase in risky behavior?

In answer, they highlight research by Dr. Garcia and Dr. Reiber that places blame with **pluralistic ignorance (PI)**.

PI: the phenomenon that describes people when they behave in ways that go against their own beliefs; when they think that

> the group's beliefs that they want to belong to are different from their own.

In other words, college students want to be in the "cool crowd" and are afraid they will be excluded if they don't participate in hookup culture. Dr. Garcia and Dr. Reiber did their research at a mid-sized public university where, sure enough, 81 percent of over 500 students said that they had hooked up. When asked about their comfort level with the hookup(s), they found, in agreement with previous research, that men had a higher level of comfort with all hookup behavior than women. Additionally, men overestimated women's comfort levels with both oral and vaginal sex, which holds more potential risk for women than for men—STDs, unintended pregnancy, etc. It was also discovered that PI affected students' perceptions of their own genders. They thought that other members of the same sex were more comfortable with hookups than they actually were.

Women in particular were more likely to be uncomfortable with hookup sex acts, but many of them participated anyway.[177] Recently, I had a conversation with a former student who is now a Student Life professional herself at a college in the US. As an undergraduate herself, she was a member of a sorority and shared that she and her sorority sisters often sat around and asked each other why they let guys get away with treating them like they did. This young woman admitted that under hookup culture they didn't really feel that they had any other choice and felt that the concept and lifestyle *Battles of the Sexes* presents would ideally offer a new and better alternative, especially for college women.

We hope it will do just that.

That same young lady also shared that in the last month alone three young women had come to her office to talk with her about negative issues related to hookup culture. Knowing what we do, we believe that many of these hookup-related sexual insults and sexual assaults can be prevented, and young women can and should enjoy their college years in happiness and safety.

We have to promote doing what you believe in as the new norm, rather than perpetuating hookup culture and the idea that following the pathway we mistakenly think everyone else is on is the right course of action..

Dr. Garcia, Dr. Reiber, and Dr. Helen Fisher may put it best when they say that findings show a majority of both college women and college men who are motivated to take part in hookups, but many times desire a more romantic relationship, are consistent with a nuanced perspective that takes into account changing social expectations, new developmental patterns, and the cross-cultural and biological importance of the pair bond.

We advocate for an even stronger movement away from hookup culture during your college years.

This romance movement may already be started across Western society. The decade-old website, OKCupid.com, has been asking their customers personal preference questions since the site first started. The trend has been moving steadily towards more celebrity risqué behavior, instant porn sites, and an overall sex-saturated media where hookups are portrayed as the norm. Meanwhile, understandably and consequently, STD rates have also been skyrocketing.[178] Research by the CDC has shown that the combined total cases of gonorrhea, chlamydia, and syphilis reached an unprecedented high in 2015. The 15-24 age group made up 53 percent of the gonorrhea cases and 65 percent of the cases of chlamydia.[179] In 2013, the CDC declared STDs a severe epidemic and HPV as the primary driver of it. Presently the CDC considers HPV to be the most commom STD in America. Women and men both gert HPV, but the longterm effects are much more dangerous for women. The American Cancer society considers

HPV to be *the* cause of cervical cancer. As a matter of fact, women are 125 percent more likely than men to have HPV develop into cancer. Women bear a disproportionate load of STDs overall. The CDC flatly stated that a female's anatomy can place her at unique risk for STD infection in comparison to a male.[180] Danger and damage done to college women notwithstanding, when it comes to sexual behavior and values, there seems to have been more and more of the attitude that anything goes.

At least until 2016.

In 2016, OKCupid.com users' personal preferences began to change as the site continued asking the same questions. The answers to two particular queries were the most telling. One asked, "Would you consider sleeping with someone on the first date?" Compared to 2005, *every single demographic group* was more likely to say no. Straight women led the pack with 25 percent being less likely to say yes. When they were asked, "Would you date someone just for sex?" again, every demographic group said no more than in 2005. There was an overall decline of 10 percent.[181]

Along those same lines, a large US national research study of over 3,000 young adults and high school students was released in 2017 by Harvard University. It found that a large majority of young adults are overestimating how many other young people are hooking up (which agrees with Reiber and Garcia's research on PI). They also discovered that 85 percent of young adults would prefer other options over hooking up, such as hanging out with friends or having sex within a committed relationship. The study agrees with Garcia and Reiber, who say that when this overestimation occurs, young people can feel ashamed or embarrassed to not be a part of the casual sex scene they perceive as the norm.[182]

These research findings are a step in the right direction, and we want to be part of a romantic renaissance. We encourage young people, especially young women, to think carefully about this whole situation and culture and consider joining the back-to-romance movement.

Back to Biology

Under the hookup culture, there are many more problems besides the ones we've already addressed. A recent article in the Journal of College Student Psychotherapy showed that data analysis of 72,067 college students reveals that stalking, physical abuse, emotional abuse, and relationship difficulties in general are very common.[183] Clearly, the relational environment on college campuses is broken and needs to be fixed.

One of the reasons that young women may be able to better see the true situation and do something about it is that the female brain is significantly different from males (but you knew that already). Barbara Annis and Keith Merron outline some of these differences. One of the most obvious differences is the size of the corpus callosum, which has a large effect on how humans process information. It is now common knowledge that the brain is divided into hemispheres. The left brain is the seat of logical and linear thought. The right brain is the base for holistic, creative, and intuitive thinking. The corpus callosum connects the two halves. With the corpus callosum being larger in women's brains, it allows them to engage in right-brain and left-brain activities *at the same time*. Because of this size difference, men can seem to have a one-track mind at times in comparison to women. The size and shape of a woman's corpus callosum also helps decipher things like unspoken parts of a meeting or exchange, such as body language, vocal tone, and facial expression, while simultaneously staying engaged in the present moment.

Another important difference in women and men's brains is in the anterior cortex. Women have a larger anterior cortex, which allows them to integrate and arrange memories and emotions into more complex patterns of thought compared to men.[184] As a result, women have the tendency to weigh more variables, consider more options, and are able to see a wider assortment of solutions to problems than men typically do. This difference in the anterior cortex makes possible women's greater sensitivity to gut instinct and is considered to be the seat of "women's intuition."

Yet another important area of difference is the insular cortex. This organ is very complex and influences our emotional response to our environment. It helps control our heartbeat and blood pressure and affects basic functions like swallowing and speaking, and is also involved in our consciousness and sense of self. It regulates our sense of pain, along with heat and cold, and orders our responses to external stimuli, creating feelings such as disgust or empathy. The insular cortex is twice as large on average in women's brains than it is in men's. This helps them to translate unconscious thoughts into conscious thoughts that are often greatly affected by memories and emotions. The insular cortex allows women to draw more on past experiences and learn from them, preventing them from acting in haste and taking unnecessary risks compared to men.

Is any of this sounding familiar?

The hippocampus is yet another brain area that has sex differences.[185] It too is larger and much more active in the female brain and can help explain why women are usually better at expressing their emotions and remembering intricate details of events from the past.[186] Having a larger hippocampus is one of the factors explaining why women benefit so much by talking through their problems. Being able to better access and freely express their emotions helps women deal more effectively with stress. This larger hippocampus can also help women efficiently process and code emotional experiences into long-term memory. Oftentimes, women have richer and more intense memories of emotional events than men.[187]

The last sex difference of the brain that I'll point out from Annis and Merron's work (although they describe many more) is in the prefrontal cortex. If it appears that girls mature more quickly than boys, it's because they do. The prefrontal cortex, which is the part of the brain that is in charge of judgement, decision making, and willpower, is both larger and quicker to develop in girls than in boys.[188] The prefrontal cortex is in charge of executive function and is the seat of the ability to decide which course of action might be bad, better, or best. Importantly, as the judgement center of the brain, it regulates and controls social behavior by moderating the actions of the more reactive amygdala (which, as we discussed in earlier chapters, is the brain's primitive survival, command, and control center). Have you ever noticed that males tend to be more exploratory, impulsive, and risk-taking than females? This difference is a big part of the reason why.[189]

Additionally, Dr. Larry Cahill, an eminent neuroscientist at the University of California, Irvine, has outlined the research on sex differences in animals that he states create brain influences on all levels. These include sex difference influences all the way down to the molecular and ion-channel levels. He says that the brains of mammals are overflowing with differences that cannot be explained by human culture and that the animal reaserch proves that the human mammalian brain must contain all kinds of biologically-based differences that cannot be explained simply by human culture. He goes on to highlight human research that highlights sex difference influennces on behavior through human brain structure and human brain genetics.[190]

So why did we just go through all of those differences?

These sex differences should make clear that men and women have very different ways of processing information in certain situations. Yet another very recent large-scale study by Dr. Daniel Amen compared 46,034 SPECT (single photon emission computed tomography) imaging studies calculating the differences between the brains of men and women. He found that the brains of women were significantly more active than the brains of men. This is particularly true in the prefrontal cortex and limbic areas of the brain.[191]

We hope that by understanding these differences and keeping them in mind, you can escape hookup culture and so many of the other destructive elements of college life (substance abuse, cutting, etc.) and have a positive and healthy undergraduate experience.

We hope that this knowledge can be helpful in the prevention of heartbreak and heartache.

The Ounce of Prevention

Since this might be your last piece of (somewhat) formalized relationship education, we wanted to end this chapter with some preventive self-knowledge for you.

Once again, remember that studies have shown that women's reproductive-related hormones vary considerably during the monthly twenty-eight-day menstrual cycle.[192] As estrogen starts to surge on the eighth or ninth day, it promotes ovulation. This corresponds with a five-day window of fertility that ends on the day of ovulation.[193] At the same time as estrogen surges, so does testosterone, and this contributes to women's increased sexual desires.[194] Women's ratings of men's attractiveness change over the course of the menstrual cycle and as you approach the fertile window each month, your preference in type of mate may shift.[195] Research has shown that during the time of high fertility, you may find yourself more attentive to physically attractive men[196] and you may be more aroused by sexually explicit materials.[197] During this time, you may be more attracted to taller men, the scents of men with symmetrical body features,[198] more masculine faces, deeper voices,[199] dominant behavior patterns, and a generally dominant personality.

All of these traits, plus a body with a waist-to-hip ratio of about 0.8 or 0.9 (which means that the man's waist is 80 percent to 90 percent of his hip measurement), and waist-to-chest ratio of about 0.7 (waist being 70 percent the size of the chest), women find very attractive. In other words, women have the tendency to be attracted to men with a muscular (but not too muscular) V-shape. All of this is especially true during the fertile window each month. This presents potential problems to marriages, especially if the woman is married to a less physically attractive man.[200] Research has found that women's desire for masculine faces is directly related to their estrogen levels.[201] Women with higher circulating levels of estrogen have a stronger preference for masculine faces. During the lower fertility portion of your cycle, your preference for these masculine physical and behavioral characteristics declines and your desire for characteristics such as emotional sensitivity and nurturing traits that characterize a good father increase.[202]

You might be asking, "What does this have to do with me? I'm a college (or young) woman with my mind on other things."

The years from now until the average age of first marriage for American women, which is 27, will fly by. You need a heads up on these important matters. Currently, around 85-90 percent of men and women in the US are projected to be married.[203] There is obviously a better chance that you will be in the 85-90 percent of those that do marry (if you're not already) than the 10-15 percent of those that don't. If you're like most women, when you go to practice your female choice, you'll have to choose between maybe a hotter bad-boy type versus one that may be physically less desirable, but more desirable as a good, loyal husband and devoted father. I hate to break it to you, but there are very few highly masculine, tall, dark and handsome, dominant, and creative hunks who are also loyal husbands and devoted fathers. If you find one, great. But the odds are not in your favor.

Women have had to make mating decisions based on trade-offs between genetic fitness and male fidelity, combined with resource-providing capability, for quite some time. Many choose in favor of what will benefit their future children, whether consciously or unconsciously. I've warned young men throughout other parts of this book about their inherited genetic tendencies to ruin their most important relationship through infidelity. I'm doing the same now for young women. Be aware of your tendency for fertile folly.

Another thing to keep in mind is a phenomenon Dr. Judith Easton and her colleagues at the University of Texas uncovered. They found in their research that women, starting in their late 20s, think more about sex, have more frequent and intense sexual fantasies, and take part in sexual intercourse more often than women in other age groups, *including college women*.[204] In other words, your sexual peak is still ahead of you if you are a college woman reading this. The researchers hypothesize that happens because of women's declining fertility during that time, and that women are motivated unconsciously by their ticking biological clock to do something about it. Be armed with this knowledge to avoid situations that can wreck your romance with the true love of your life. Of particular concern are occasions that involve alcohol. Even a little bit causes an increase in women's testosterone levels and may make many of you more sexually aggressive. In men, it actually makes testosterone levels drop, but as you know, young men usually have such an overabundance that the drop doesn't affect them much. The threat to women's fidelity comes especially when alcohol is consumed during the fertile window.[205] In this state, women may become as sexually irresponsible and aggressive as men in their natural state. That can be a recipe for romance disaster for you and the love of your life.

Romance Renaissance

We believe, with the execution of this knowledge, there can be a new romantic renaissance movement among young adults in Western societies. This is what we stand for and we're unafraid, unashamed, and unapologetic for being romance advocates. And we hope you will join us!

So, what do we have to gain from following this pathway?

Dr. Susan Pinker lays out the benefits of marriage. Married people enjoy stronger and more stable relationships and superior physical and psychological wellness. Far fewer married couples are depressed or alcoholics. They live longer and happier lives despite coming from all kinds of different backgrounds. This is true in almost all Western societies no matter how liberal or conservative the culture. A study that took place in the late 1990s showed that in seventeen Westernized industrial nations, including Canada, the UK, and most of Europe, married couples were significantly happier than those who simply lived together. Also, couples who live together are happier than single and divorced people. It seems that the closer we are to a married state, the better and happier our lives are. That is the romantic love we are recommending and it's clear that it is one of the best steps humans can take to increase our well-being.[206]

A Word from Sarah

We have a better understanding now about how our female nature affects our behaviors and clashes with Western culture. How can we make these aspects of our nature work for us instead of against us? Here are a few ways I've found to be helpful:

- *Mindfulness*
- *Adjusting our schedule to allow for regular physical activity*

- *Satisfying cravings for sweet foods with living foods that naturally contain sugar (fruits)*
- *Satisfying cravings for fat-heavy foods with living foods that naturally contain healthy fats (avocado, nuts, seeds)*
- *Carving out time on a regular basis to plan meals and snacks to avoid last-minute, drive-thru binges*
- *Eating out rarely, or simply making better choices when we do, seeking out unprocessed, living foods*
- *Weigh or take measurements regularly to identify when excess weight begins to creep on and prevent further weight gain*

Having been through college, marriage, and childbearing while working full time, starting a business, and dealing with significant medical issues, I know it's hard to find the time and energy to make these decisions on a regular basis.

*What I can tell you is **it's worth it**.*

───────────── A SARAH SUMMARY: ─────────────

- Young women are unfortunately more prone to depression, anxiety, low self-esteem, guilt, and general overwhelm.
- A combination of the decreased age of puberty, later marriage, a desire to fit in, and an increase in Western hookup culture creates a mismatch between the biological norm for a woman's reproductive nature and her reality. For women, knowing traits to watch out for and staying mindful of the detriments of alcohol and hookup culture can help avoid some of the negative psychological reactions we are more prone to and increase our chances of finding lasting love.

Chapter 11

· · · · · · · · · ·

Romance Wreckers—An Ounce of Prevention for Him

"Hogamous, Higamous, Man is Polygamous,
Higamous, Hogamous, Woman is Monogamous"
DOROTHY PARKER

Man to Man

In this chapter, I am writing to young men and college men in particular, but I am also writing to myself. We are all in the same boat. This Testosterone Trap situation has the potential for disastrous effects on all of our lives. I've found that learning about the biological forces on the inside can be greatly helpful to us men in understanding how to control these genetically encoded tendencies we have inherited. I know it has made a huge difference in my life and I want you to learn these things early in order to avoid heartache and loss.

Why do women seem to be monogamous and men seem to be polygamous?

In *How Pleasure Works*, Paul Bloom outlines the situation. Our developmental history is evidenced in our bodies. Size differences between the sexes reflect the level of competition between males that is necessary for them to be able to mate with as many females as possible. The size difference is also related to the level of effort that the two sexes put into parenting with the smaller sex usually being the one that puts the most effort into parenting.[207] Human males, on average, are about 20 percent bigger than females. Our size difference, or more technically stated sexual dimorphism, is significant but not as large as some species. This reflects a moderate level of polygyny, which means, in some cases, one man would have been with several women.[208]

In a polygynous society, some men (often the bigger, stronger ones) end up with many wives. Some end up with one (monogamy) and some end up with none. Our ancestral environment, with a gender ratio birthrate that was around 50 percent, became a feast or famine situation. For high-testosterone men, there were plenty of women and their genes became over-represented in future generations. For other men, there was just one woman and, in some cases, this proved very effective for getting their genes represented in future generations because they were very successful in taking care of their kids and making them great parents themselves. But for many men, there were no wives; therefore, women became a scarce resource. Hopefully, you see that in the succeeding tens of thousands of generations, men having access to sex with women became a very big deal indeed in our species' genetic encoding process!

Paul Bloom concurs and writes that our developmental history became embodied in our male psychology. We males on average are more interested in sex with multiple partners.[209] In *Do Gentlemen Really Prefer Blondes*, Gena Pincott quotes research that shows that one in four males worldwide would prefer to have more than one sexual partner per month.[210] For comparison purposes, only one in thirty-three American women say they would want to have more than one sexual partner in a month. The smallest gap between women and men are between women and men in Eastern Europe, where one in thirteen women say they would prefer more than one sexual partner per month.

No doubt the Coolidge effect is at work here.

Coolidge effect: A very common effect among mammals. Male rats, rams, cows, and sheep all display it. In studies, for instance, a cow is placed in a bullpen and after sex the cow is replaced by another cow. The bull's sexual response goes on and on with each new cow presented, but quickly disappears if the cow he has already copulated with is left in the pen. He never wants seconds from an earlier sexual conquest. However, males do continue to be aroused and able to ejaculate in response to novel females. The arousal reaction with up to the twelfth novel female was nearly as powerful as it had been to the first.

Researchers also experimented with rams and ewes and found the same general reaction. They even tried to disguise an ewe with a covering of a canvas tarp with whom the ram had already had sex and introducing her as a novel female, but they could never successfully fool the ram. They found that the reduced arousal did not have to do with the ewe already having sex because when they brought in ewes that had copulated with other rams, the ram who had not copulated with her still responded enthusiastically. Arousal went down only when the ewe was one the ram had already personally mated with.[211]

What does this say to us men?

Animal House

We need to be aware that we too may share some of these animalistic tendencies to be drawn to novel sex partners and, in the process, betray the love of our life.

With the Coolidge effect in mind, it is not hard to see why men are also more aroused by and interested in casual sex with anonymous people. This is true worldwide, as sex difference research has been carried out cross-culturally. Prostitution has come into existence mostly to address this male desire for variety, and this is also true for the pornography industry. There are male sex workers and male eroticism and nakedness that is portrayed in pornography, but this is mostly to cater to the desires of gay men.[212]

Paul Bloom gets to the heart of the matter when he writes:

> "One consideration is that human children are particularly fragile creatures, born far too early with a long period of dependence on adults for food and shelter and protection from predators, both animal and human. Fathers matter, then, as they help in protecting and raising the children (and also because they protect the mother) because if she dies while the baby is feeding, the baby is likely to die too... This does not mean that mothers and fathers are interchangeable. That remains an evolutionary battle of the sexes because it is in the male's genetic interest to fool around on the side. This would be bad news for the female, who would be better off with a mate who sticks with her and her child(ren) instead of distributing his time and resources to other offspring and women... This conflict shapes female preferences about who to mate with. They are looking for males who show signs of future fidelity. Men might evolve to fake these signs, but if women are good at seeing through this deception, then males

who tend to be sexually and romantically faithful might out-produce the cads. It is attractive, then, to be faithful. In this way, sexual selection will serve to narrow the gap between men and women's sexual preferences."[213]

Narrow the Gap

We stand fully behind the narrowing of that gap and want to use any and all means to help young men and women accomplish it. In my experience, one of the major ways this can be accomplished is to learn to better understand ourselves and the inherited biochemical processes behind our motivations.

We now turn to Paul Zak again, whose work we focused on earlier with young women and oxytocin. We've established that there is a tradeoff between testosterone and oxytocin in human behavior and that females and males have disproportionate amounts of each. This sex difference is pretty pronounced with testosterone being heavily weighted in men's direction. Testosterone makes men do strange things. It is this hormone that motivates men's risk taking, the inordinate amount of male violence, and the male species hallmark behavior, the reckless pursuit of intercourse regardless of the consequences. This hormonal mismatch has led to the parade of male-based sex scandals over the years. From Bill Clinton to Tiger Woods, male after male has fallen into The Testosterone Trap.

Of course, testosterone does have its positive aspects. For example, it elevates athletic performance because it increases muscle percentages and bone density. It also is very helpful for people like emergency responders, who at times must display overt risk with physical courage, raw strength, and speed. This was also proven important and valuable for our ancestors when threatening animals had to be fought off. As time went on, we had to go further and begin to hunt threatening animals for meat. We also needed to be able to lift and otherwise labor to control our environment better. Also, it wasn't only the animals that were threatening to our hunting and gathering ancestors. Living in bands of 100-150 and constantly roaming in search of food meant that you were running into other bands of humans from time to time. Having big, menacing, high-testosterone males as part of your band meant there was a good chance that the other bands would leave you alone. The main reason that high testosterone was evolutionarily selected was that it made sure those genes made it into future generations in high numbers. And the ability of high-testosterone males to out-compete other males for the chance to mate, again, with as many females as possible certainly helped with that selection.

> Men mating with as many females as possible means that far fewer men than women make up our ancestors. DNA markers show that a single male, again possibly Genghis Khan, had 500 wives and 500 concubines and is a direct male ancestor of .05 percent of the world's population of males (or around 16 million). The fathering champion in purely numerical terms was a man named Ismail who sired a record 888 children. For comparison purposes, the numerical mothering champion was a Russian woman who had a record sixty-nine children, mostly through multiple births.

Over millions of years of development, there emerged a two-way method of species survival. Both genders were potentially capable of violence, being competitive, and being aggressive. But the high-testosterone men were more hormonally predisposed to carry out that role. At the same time, both genders were capable of bonding, compassion, and nurturing, but the high-oxytocin females were hormonally predisposed for taking the lead in that area.

Before we talk further about the extensive downsides of too much testosterone, there is one more positive outcome to high levels of testosterone. From time to time, there are certain individuals in society who do not play by the rules and break the law. Research has shown that high-testosterone individuals are more willing to dole out punishment than low-testosterone ones. The tendency for punishing the bad guy is further supported by activation of the dopamine reward pathway for males much more than for females. Research has shown that societies that promote positive behavior by not only rewarding the good, but also punishing the bad, have the best results.[214]

A Violent Mix

It's important to point out that most crimes are carried out by young men, and the majority of murderers are males between 20-25 years old. David Geary writes, "There is no known society which has levels of violence among females that can even come close to those of males."

In a study of same sex murders that was cross-cultural and went back more than 700 years, it was found that male-on-male murder occurred at a rate that was thirty to forty times the rate of female-on-female murder. Male-on-male murder happened most frequently during the initial mate selection part of life, which occurs from the late teens through the early twenties. It is more common among unmarried men. On the same note, around two thirds of male-on-male murders happen as a result of social disputes rather than a crime such as a robbery. Over half of those homicides are related to status, competition, and saving face.[215]

Dr. David P. Barash makes the excellent point in *Out of Eden* that the mismatch between our genetically encoded nature and our technologically advanced society creates another battle of the sexes. He insightfully points out that the history of "civilization" is one of human's incessant advancements in the ability to kill with increasing ease at greater and greater distances and in ever-increasing numbers. Dr. Barash cites the evolution from club, knife, and spear to musket, rifle, cannon, machine gun, battleship, bomber, and missile-delivered nuclear weapons. While all of this lethal technological progress has been made, the humans controlling the weapons have not changed at all. Biologically, we are weak and poorly designed to kill compared to other creatures. We don't have the teeth, claws, or jaws other animals are equipped with. Using only our natural equipment, we would find it tough to kill another single human, let alone hundreds of millions. But our cultural progress has changed all that.

Creatures who do come equipped with lethal weaponry—like eagles, cougars, lions, and alligators—are not inclined to use them against members of their own species. If they did, it would hurt their chances of species survival over countless generations. We humans on the other hand have not developed these same instincts when it comes to our own kind. Dr. Barash points out that this is one of the reasons guns can be so dangerous in our society. And I would add that they are much more so in the hands of young men. He says that the lethal consequences of one small movement—putting a few ounces of pressure on a trigger—is magnified by superb technology into violence that has dreadful results. In contrast, if we had to live or die by the use of direct biological force alone, there would be a whole lot more living and a whole lot less dying.[216] This genetic-cultural mismatch makes the mission of human males getting a better handle on their own reproductive, nature-inspired emotions a very high priority indeed!

Men also murder women more than women kill men. Much of this killing and wife beating is rooted in mate guarding and sexual jealousy. While these behaviors may have been reproductively advantageous during the Paleolithic, they were still ethically wrong then and they certainly don't fit into a positive, twenty-first century society.

Testosterone Poisoning

Paul Zak says that adolescent and young adult men can be considered to be suffering from "testosterone poisoning" during the initial reproductive competition stage of their life. This Testosterone Trap, as we call it, can lead to many regrettable decisions, especially in the arena of committed relationships.[217] Rats who have similar physiology and brain systems to ours can once again be illustrative of our challenges as men. In another study which showcased the Coolidge effect, male rats' dopamine was shown to rise in response to a new and different female, even though he had recently been sexually satiated.[218] This mechanism works in a similar manner in human male brains as well, which is obviously a challenge to men's fidelity in committed relationships. The bad news is that testosterone levels peak in the late teens and early 20s and only start slowly declining in men after they reach 30 years old.

The question is, what can we do about it?

Fighting the Testosterone Trap

It turns out that there are lots of things we can do to fight this "testosterone poisoning." First of all, because of inherited genetics, if we are in a committed relationship, we should consider ourselves to be in a kind of addictive situation. Just as an alcoholic avoids bars, we should learn to avoid certain tempting venues. We can identify these by the reactions taking place between people in what we call "chemical cocktail parties." The first place we should be wary of as college students is literally at parties. If we are working in an office, this can also threaten relationships. Over 60 percent of affairs begin as office romances. Business travel is another arena where there are particular challenges to fidelity for men.

Basically, anywhere alcohol is served, or where other drugs are being taken, is especially risky. Remember that alcohol raises women's testosterone levels and lowers the inhibitory action of their frontal lobe. It also lowers *your* frontal lobe's ability to help maintain control in tempting situations.

The Trade-Off of Serontonin and Dopamine

We can be proactive with our lifestyles. Serotonin and dopamine are in a trade-off relationship, so if serotonin goes up, it forces dopamine to go down. And dopamine is the hormone that drives sexual arousal. There are many ways we can raise serotonin naturally, and we should take advantage of that knowledge. For instance, aerobic exercise raises serotonin levels. In fact, any kind of sustained muscular movement, even something as small as gum chewing, can raise serotonin levels. Another natural serotonin raiser is sun exposure. If you make a habit of getting out into the sun in the morning and throughout the day, it will also help. You don't even have to actually be in the sun to get the serotonin-raising effect. All that is necessary is for bright light to be seen and go through the optic chiasm back to the pineal body in the the brain.

Certain foods also have an effect on dopamine and noradrenaline levels in the mind and body. High-protein foods have the tendency to raise dopamine and noradrenaline since they are primarily made from amino acids, while carbohydrates have the tendency to raise levels of serotonin (although too many carboyhydrates, especially if they are refined, simple, and starchy, and eaten without accompanying protein and fat, can promote excess body fat). By exercising and eating a balanced diet, you can maintain high levels of serotonin. For progressive relaxation, meditation and exercise like yoga can also lower cortisol levels. Cortisol also has an inverse relationship with serotonin, so by lowering cortisol, you help raise serotonin. Speaking of cortisol, it is raised by stimulants such as coffee, soda, candy bars, and other caffeine-containing foods. It is good to minimize these if we are looking to raise serotonin.

To add further insight to the dopamine-serotonin inverse relationship when it comes to sex, let me share an experience that I had when one of the ladies from my Women's Personal Conditioning class approached me for help with a problem. She took me aside after class one day and told me she was struggling with something. I immediately told her, as I do with all of my students, that I would be glad to help if I could. She then proceeded to shock me with the revelation that she was having problems with her boyfriend because she had lost her sex drive. It took me by surprise but I didn't let on and as I thought about it I was humbled and grateful that she trusted me enough to bring her challenging situation to me in this way.

I began by thinking of my own past experiences with depression and anti-depressant medication. I asked her if she was on any SSRIs (Selective Serotonin Reuptake Inhibitors) and, sure enough, she was. From research and experience I knew personally that raising brain levels of serotonin lowered libido. I also asked if she would happen to be on hormonal birth control and she answered yes again. These also lower women's sex drive. When we remember that women on average have much less testosterone and dopamine than men in the first place, it is not surprising that lowered libido is becoming a bigger and bigger challenge to many women in Western societies. With this new-found knowledge and in consultation with her doctor, she was able to normalize her sex drive by the end of the semester. She even volunteered to share her experiences with her classmates on the final day of class. The thought I took away from her situation was that if this was happening to a healthy and fit college student, how many more women in Western societies was it happening to and would they ever tell anybody and ask for help? It is something we will probably see more and more of in the future. In many ways, some twenty-first century Western women have just the opposite challenge that men do: not enough testosterone with raised levels of serotonin not helping the problem.

Strategy

The other big moderator of the behavioral effects of testosterone is oxytocin. Paul Zak recommends for everyone to have at least eight hugs a day. Every time a hug occurs, both party's oxytocin levels go up.

Another tactic to employ in a tempting situation is mentally reframing the situation, which can help testosterone levels go down. This can be a substantial exercise, as testosterone levels can rise as much as 30 percent in men when we are turned on. I counsel the men I work with to try to reframe a situation where they are attracted to a committed woman (or are themselves committed) by thinking of that woman as a wonderful work of art. If that doesn't help, I encourage them to think of her as their sister. If that doesn't work, I tell them to get outta Dodge, because the limbic-system-based temptation will probably win in the end.

Oxytocin is also raised when we commit ourselves to a woman and really mean it. If we are fortunate enough to have children, testosterone declines even more and oxytocin is raised in its place. One note of caution here though. In recent research, it has been shown that because of the strong bonds between oxytocin and vasopressin, which is a similar male analog to oxytocin, men can sometimes become dangerous if a marriage is threatened once it is established. Vasopressin is a more territorial oxytocin-like hormone that makes male mammals mark their territories. If their territory is threatened, even from within, males can sometimes react with violence.

Zak, being the expert on oxytocin and its relationship to testosterone, laughs about purposefully trying to become more of a girly-man by spending time brushing his daughters' hair and helping pick out dresses for them. He says he couldn't have imagined himself doing this in his younger years when he was into playing football and working on cars. He reports that he takes fewer risks, gets into fewer arguments and fights with men, and is a more careful driver now. He believes that he has become much more tolerant and forgiving, saying that this greater ability to have empathy and nurture his children will do wonders to help them develop their own set of robust oxytocin receptors. This loving attention will help them bestow the same benefit on their own children someday.[219]

I have to agree wholeheartedly. I've had the same experiences in my life as my consciousness has been raised to their importance. In our final chapter, we will give even more oxytocin-promoting personal advice, particularly focused on that crucial relationship you have with your very special someone.

Pass the Monogomy, Please

But first, is a happy marriage even feasible in twenty-first century, Western societies?

An authority on the subject, biological anthropologist Dr. Helen Fisher, seems to think so. She concedes that many anthropologists believe that because so many societies permit polygyny, creating harems is the badge of the human animal. Dr. Fisher is not among them and thinks that polygyny is an opportunistic mating strategy. She says that in most of the societies where polygyny is permitted, only about 5-10 percent of males actually have several wives simultaneously. Even though polygyny is broadly discussed, in reality it is practiced on a much smaller scale. Instead, the large majority of almost every society in the world forms a pair-bond with serial monogamy being the most common reproductive pattern.

For further proof, she cites George Peter Murdock, who after surveying 250 human cultures summarized by saying that an impartial observer using numerical preponderance as their yardstick would be forced to characterize nearly every known human society as monogamous, despite the preference for and frequency of the practice of polygyny in the overwhelming majority. Because human polygyny has been associated with hierarchy and wealth, monogamy was very likely more prevalent throughout our two-million-year hunting and gathering past.[220] I would tend to agree that despite our inherent polygynous tendency-related difficulties, in practical terms, most of humanity's relational past has been defined by monogamous, romantic love relationships.

--------------------- A SARAH SUMMARY: ---------------------

- Men are unique in that, based on the Coolidge effect, they are aroused by novelty and are more prone to seek multiple partners and stray from a monogamous partnership.
- A hallmark of the male species: the reckless pursuit of intercourse regardless of the consequences due to this behavior being genetically in the man's favor over the years of evolution.
- Raising serotonin and lowering cortisol naturally can help with controlling testosterone's negative effects such as aerobic activity, sun exposure, eating a balanced diet, meditation, and limiting stimulants.

Chapter 12

• • • • • • • • • •

United We Stand, Romantically Ever After

"We are most free from biological constraints in
proportion to our understanding of those inclinations and
predispositions with which evolution has endowed us."
DAVID P. BARASH

"And ye shall know the truth,
and the truth shall make you free."
JESUS

United and Understood

would like to start our final chapter on this journey of self-discovery
and self-understanding with another profoundly impactful personal
experience.

After I had finished a SEX IQ presentation at a Greek organization
at a large university, a student approached me. This young adult

related how what had been taught struck very close to home for them and that they knew from personal experience what I meant when I taught The Testosterone Trap. They said that their dad had left their mom and the three siblings when they were young children for a younger woman. Of course, it crushed the innocent mom who, as often happens, was blindsided by her husband's infidelity. The four of them couldn't understand why he would leave all of them for this new, younger woman. It was heartbreaking to see the look of anguish on this college student's face as the terrible memories were shared. This young person said that because of SEX IQ they now understood what was going on and that it was helpful. While the understanding itself couldn't fix anything, it did bring some peace of mind. It wasn't their fault. It was their father's fault and the mismatched sexual chemistry involved that no one understood at the time, not even him. I could see that the SEX IQ presentation was helping to bring closure to one of the most traumatic chapters of this Millennial's life.

That experience burned a place in my memory. Here were the traumatizing consequences and bitter fruit of a lack of understanding of his own human reproductive nature by a husband and father. I realized in that moment that there were millions of other young adults out there who, unfortunately, had similar life experiences. I came to also understand that infidelity, at 37 percent of cases,[221] is most often the cause of divorce in the US. At that point, a strong resolve began to grow in me that these biologically-driven, motivational insights and knowledge of our human sexual nature *must* be shared widely to young adults throughout Western societies to prevent history from repeating itself. It has become our major mission to prevent such heartbreak.

As a part of that mission, it has been the goal of *Battles of the Sexes* to bring greater understanding of these inclinations and predispositions women and men have inherited that behaviorally affect our present-day population. This final chapter attempts to shed even more light on these battles of the sexes.

To be clear, there is an inborn sexual conflict of interest between women and men. In *Sex at Dusk*, Lynn Saxon writes that the joint project of reproduction can mask conflict between women and men. Males potentially have more to gain from any one act of sex (fertilizing eggs with potentially no cost) and much more to lose from not mating (possibly missing the only chance for impregnation that is coming his way). As a result, men have been selected for eager and persistent sexuality traits and women have been selected for choosy and resistant sexuality traits.

In looking across nature, there are some species where males try to influence and coerce female choice in ways that can harm the female's lifelong reproductive capability. Again, sexual conflict is essentially the conflict between, over, if, when, and how often to mate, because the two sexes have different naturally-selected optimal behaviors.

Sexual Peace

Research on natural and sexual selection is often done using fruit flies because of their very short life span. Remember the experiment from earlier (page 110)?

Although the previous experiment wasn't the most positive, there is good news. The good news is that other experiments were done where monogamy was mandated on the flies. In this situation, the reproductive interests of both sexes joined forces on the same offspring and the male's sperm competition was ended. The semen became less and less harmful to the females. Also, the males developed less aggression in their courtship behaviors and reproductive output was higher than it had been with sperm competition. In repeated experiments, it was found that it took only forty-seven generations of monogamy to bring the same improvements in the males. This is of monumental importance and is what *Battles of the Sexes* is all about.

It seems that monogamy over time brings sexual peace where there was once sexual conflict.

Lynn Saxon says, "Only with lifetime sexual monogamy can the interest of both parents converge on the very same offspring and extend together for both the parent's lifetimes so that what harms the reproductive fitness of one sex harms that of the other too and is therefore not selected" (*Sex at Dusk,* page 27).[222]

Dr. Sarah Blaffer Hrdy agrees, "If such a thing [such as enforced monogamy] could be imposed on other species including humans, there is no reason to think that a similar result could not be obtained and the priority of both men and women would be the well-being of children."

Hrdy goes on to write that monogamy turns out to be an exceptionally solid reproductive style because it raises the survival chances of the offspring. It lowers the ingrained conflicts of interest between the sexes and over extended periods of time, sexual monogamy becomes the cure-all for various kinds of detrimental devices that one sex uses to exploit the other.[223]

While this is great news, there is a big challenge that goes along with it. As we have seen previously, many young men are driven to try to have multiple sex partners. These drives are embedded in the unconscious mind. Dr. David Buss points out how the unconscious mind works. Take our sweat glands, for example, which help with the thermal regulation of our bodies. We don't need to think about them in a hot situation; they activate automatically through the power of our unconscious minds as the body's natural response.[224]

Can you imagine trying to make yourself consciously stop sweating?

In a heated sexual situation, our unconscious minds also go into automatic mode to respond to the situation. It takes some conscious effort to counteract it, and often a great deal of willpower!

That is what *Battles of the Sexes* is all about—empowering young men and women to obtain the self-knowledge which enables them to gain self-mastery, especially with regard to addictive sexual and food behaviors. Barash has much to say on this entire topic.[225] He was interviewed by Laura Yan for an October 2015 blog post on "Hopes and Fears." He and other experts were asked the question, "Are humans meant to be monogamous?" His answer is quite enlightening to our understanding. He said that the truth is that people are not by nature monogamous and that monogamy is not obsolete, but rather new on the scene in human history. He cites the evidence for polygyny, some of which we have already seen: men being on average bigger than women with much more muscle mass, men being much more violence prone than women, and boys becoming sexually and socially mature at older ages than girls. He says these characteristics are true of animal species where a single male tries to mate with several females and are profoundly correlated to male-on-male competition for gaining these opportunities. The evidence from anthropologists for human polygyny is also strikingly clear, as we've seen. Around 83 percent of human societies that have not been touched by Western colonialism, and therefore have no laws against it, allow the formation of harems by men. He goes on to say that harem formation is harmful both to women and especially to the majority of men. Our species has a sex ratio that is close to equal. Therefore, with polygyny only a minority of men are mated (some with many wives), leaving most excluded and sexually frustrated. Women too suffer under the system in those societies as they may have less than optimal conditions as a result of their competition with co-wives.

And the Benefits Are...

He goes on to say that no one knows for certain how and why monogamy came to be a cultural institution mainly in the Western world, and slowly started moving out to other parts of the world.[226] We know that the Christian church around 800 AD had a role in getting monogamy through marriage embedded in the cultural fabric. Along with this, there may be the possibility of monogamy being representative of a social agreement in which powerful men who were polygynists decided to abandon their claim to exclusive access to many women in exchange for social cohesion and societal peace. There are other accounts that included the willingness of these new husbands to fight cooperatively in defense of the group. Dr. Barash goes on to agree with what other experts cited earlier in *Battles of the Sexes*.

> "Indeed, for all of the liability and strain in suppressing our biological inclinations for non-monogamy, the reality is that for human beings, monogamy offers distinct advantages as well. Notable among these is bi-parental care. In any species experiencing internal fertilization, males, but not females, are stuck with a profound biologically-mandated uncertainty. It's known as: mommy's babies, daddy's maybes. As a result, it is very rare for any to engage in bi-parental care unless the males are guaranteed confidence of their genetic relatedness to the offspring—a confidence that monogamy alone can provide. And because human children need so much parental assistance, protection, and investment, we, perhaps more than any other animals, are especially benefitted by monogamy (which incidentally need not necessarily involve individuals of two different sexes)... It is important to emphasize that even though monogamy definitely isn't natural to human beings, and therefore isn't easy, it is nonetheless possible as well as offering some important benefits. Many of humanity's most notable accomplishments—learning to play the violin, speaking multiple languages, performing delicate surgery—

are equally unnatural, but are assuredly good. They also, like successful monogamy, require hard work. It is easy to do what comes naturally. Animals do it all the time! Perhaps what makes human beings special is our ability to do things that are unnatural, whether those things are obsolete or—like monogamy—are socially imposed."[227]

So how do we imperfect human beings go about this challenging task of going against what comes naturally to us?

Knowledge is Power

Well, first and foremost, we believe in education. We have to know and understand what we are up against with our biologically-based urges and predispositions. Also, there are many holistic lifestyle practices we believe can make a major difference in gaining even more of an ability to guide and manage our human reproductive nature. One of the most important steps we can take is to give our lives a healthy base through making a wholesome and plant-based nutrition habit a cornerstone of our lifestyle. Hand in hand with this goes comprehensive, adequate exercise. This too is not easy. Dr. Lieberman says that voluntary exercise was not selected for over the millions of years of our human developmental past.[228] I try to make it a point of emphasis to teach my classes that it was not that long ago, and then stretching into the distant past, that our ancestors had no choice but to live in such a way. We have it harder in modern society in this sense than our ancestors because we have to purposely construct a physically active lifestyle. In other words, we have to be intentional and use environmental design. I give them what I call the **"grandparent rule."**

The Grandparent Rule: If your grandparents (and especially your great grandparents) did it, generally it is a good bet that I want you doing it. A couple of caveats: avoid racism and sexism, as well as smoking and chewing tobacco. A more natural lifestyle can give us the stable mind-body chemistry we need to start to make smarter sexual decisions.

Keeping in mind what we have learned about the polygynous nature of our ancestors, as time goes on in relationships, dopamine levels decrease, especially in men's brains. We have seen this Coolidge effect in various species where brain levels of dopamine are only raised when novel mates are brought into the picture.[229] Knowing this, couples should try to find ways to bring variety into their relationship. It is similar to when people eat the same foods all the time. Variety in food and sex is the spice of life, especially when it comes to sexual issues for men. Obviously, having actual new sexual partners in reality can be damaging, to say the least, to the relationship. Shared fantasy and role playing—as long as they're kept on a level of fantasy and not reality—may be a way to relieve some of the pressure and outsmart the demanding drives of our hormones. The idea is that you control the impulse to really "do it" by exploring each other's sexuality vicariously. Sensitivity should be maintained as to what is and is not acceptable to the love of your life.

Thirst for Adventure

Other dopamine-raising activities adopted by a couple may also prove to be helpful—adventures like rock climbing or whitewater rafting. It really can be any activity that you both enjoy that gets your hearts racing.

Getting back to a healthy, holistic lifestyle and getting into the habit of a disciplined and regular sleep and waking cycle means well-rested spouses who have the energy for their work life *and* sex life. Keeping electronic communication devices and their negative stimulating effects out of the bedroom is an important part of this strategy. These devices, with their sleep-inducing, melatonin-decreasing blue light and stress-producing, over-communication effects, not to mention their electromagnetic fields, can have a very damaging effect on healthy bedroom behavior. Another important thing in this realm is maintaining proper nighttime boundaries with children. It is wonderful at times to be able to snuggle with your children. It can give them a sense of safety and security. But at a certain time of night, they need to go to their own beds to sleep and give you, the parents, marital privacy.

Having mentioned stress earlier, let me say that stress management too is a very important element in keeping an active love life alive. For women especially, the presence of unsolved problems from early in the day and tensions between she and her man are going to prove very difficult to overcome. In *Unleashing the Power of the Female Brain*, Dr. Daniel Amen says women have to be able to quiet their minds from other distractions before they are able to achieve orgasms. This means keeping the stress levels down, especially in the evening. Sometimes special music can be a dopamine raiser. This will depend on the couple, but it can set a very sexy tone if done correctly.[230]

In conclusion, the intentionality that we have been talking about in regard to marriage or other long-term, committed relationships should be constantly reinforced. This isn't necessarily a dopamine raiser, but rather an oxytocin and serotonin booster. Reinforcing shared values can have a strong pair-bonding effect. When you think of your children, extended family, mutual friends, and the history you both share, it is easy to see the rarity and value of what you have together and the family you have built. Personally, I consciously and continuously work to reinforce those oxytocin-based ties. For example, I normally arise earlier than my wife and after cleaning up, I make it a habit to come back, climb up on the bed, kiss her cheek, and give her a hug before the day begins. It reminds me at the beginning of each day what I want my life to be about. Another related policy I have is that for my Facebook profile picture, I always have my wife and I pictured. It is another conscious reminder for myself and others of what I want my life to be about. It is intentional and purposeful. I also put a high priority on spending time with my children and my children's children and make it clear that family is one of my highest priorities next to my belief in God.

This is the way our parents loved each other and they set a powerful example for us to follow. My parents were married for sixty-three years before my father passed away. They are from the generation that live by the O.A.O. acronym, my "One and Only." They grew up during the Great Depression, fought World War II, and then built the US into the world's foremost industrial power. Clearly, they paid their dues in such a way that it is no wonder they are called "The Greatest Generation." Their purpose in life was to give us a better life than they had and they made that clear both through their words and their actions. They lived to impart the greater good to us kids and they demonstrated by example controlling their reproductive nature and embodying a higher form of love.

Higher Form of Love

This higher form of love was written about by a wise man named Napoleon Hill. He wrote about it way back in 1937 in one of the most bestselling books on success called *Think and Grow Rich*. In preparation for writing the book, he studied the lives of self-made men like Andrew Carnegie and Henry Ford. He found certain key things that they all did in their lives that were important to their success. One of the thirteen keys to success was something he called **sexual transmutation**.

> **Sexual transmutation:** the ability to take control of sexual energy and focus it in other positive directions. In other words, make sex serve constructive ends rather than sometimes destructive ends. One of the keys to this is finding a loving marriage partner who is complementary to the strengths and weaknesses we all have.[231]

This is the kind of self-discipline we are espousing in *Battles of the Sexes* and it can help provide the stability and dependability that often leads to great success.

Having shared spiritual beliefs is one more mightily bonding force on a couple. My wife and I are both Christians and we have always been able to look to the wisdom of the Bible for guidance. This shared belief system has helped us navigate many troubled waters in our lives. There is the satisfaction and fulfillment it brings us that makes all the hard work, and sometimes disappointments, worthwhile.

The Importance of a Family Lifestyle

Why is living the family lifestyle so important, not just for individual couples, but the species as a whole?

A family lifestyle allows for the building of attachment and trust. Susan Pinker says, "It impacts all social relationships from the bedroom to the boardroom."

She cites a 2005 study, where young men who sprayed oxytocin up their noses were more willing to hand money over to investment partners that they didn't know very well. It helped them to trust more easily and not be as worried about being ripped off.[232] I have recently realized that the success among my classes over the years I have taught has depended on this oxytocin molecule. As time has gone on, I have strived towards running the classes as a family. I set up a culture where there are lots of handshakes, pats on the back, and high fives. As a matter of fact, I have made it a point to always shake hands with each student as they enter class and often when they are leaving. I also ask them to rate how they are feeling emotionally on a scale of one to ten each day. All of these types of contact are shown to increase oxytocin levels and, of course, lower testosterone levels in turn.

Research shows that this kind of social contact decreases stress among colleagues and makes teams more cohesive. Coincidentally, each class becomes a team and gives themselves the name that they will go by for the semester. Again, semester after semester through the wonders of oxytocin, these teams have become like families. This is a crucial finding for modern societies that often succeed or fail depending on whether or not they can cooperate. If we are fortunate and come from a loving family, we get our first taste of these oxytocin-influenced psychologically-safe environments as young children growing up. It is in human ecologies such as this that great human achievements become possible. The cornerstone of all this is a loving, monogamous relationship between the parents.

One of the factors that is so beneficial about this positive environment is that it enables people to dare to dream big dreams. In *How Your Unconscious Mind Rules Your Behavior*, Dr. Leonard Mlodinow says that the psychological research literature shows over and over again that humans are benefited both personally and socially by holding positive illusions about themselves. Researchers have found that when they promote a positive mood by any means available, humans are more likely to interact with and help others. People that feel good about themselves, as Paul Zak found, are more likely to find a positive solution to their conflicts. They are better problem solvers, more determined to succeed, and more apt to persevere in the face of a challenge. This kind of positive thinking allows us to use our minds to defend against being unhappy and, by doing so, gives us the power to overcome the many obstacles in life that otherwise might overwhelm us. Research indeed shows us that humans with the most accurate self-perceptions have a tendency to be moderately depressed. Someone who has an overly positive self-evaluation is more the norm for society and is more mentally healthy.

This built-in natural human optimism is what helped our ancestors survive the tough northern European winters 50,000 years ago. It also was there when people had to experience their children dying, women dying in childbirth, and people suffering during wars, drought, flood, and famine through the eons of time. With the human experience being full of so many seemingly insurmountable barriers, nature enabled us to find a way to create an unrealistically rosy attitude about the probability of overcoming them, which is precisely what helps us do just that to this very day.[233] The end product of all of this oxytocin-based bonding, and I would contend natural human positivity, is caring for our most vulnerable population: our young.

As Dr. John Ratey and Richard Manning point out, speaking of this helpless time in human development:

> "But this topic teases out probably the most significant difference between our species and all other animals, now or ever. Our young are more or less helpless for a very long time, longer than any other species—14 or 15 years. No other species is even remotely close to us in this regard. This, too, is a defining fact of the human condition and it is not happenstance, but a predictable, derivative trait given our big brains. Humans cannot be born with fully formed brains simply because the resulting head would not fit through the birth canal. Rather, our brains are built and formed after

we are born, like a ship in a bottle. A process that takes 15, maybe 20 years."

They go on to say that this root human condition is the reason we must cooperate, and why empathy and language developed to make social cooperation possible. All of the other facets of human nature derive from this single human condition. The foundational social contract has babies as its bottom line. Ratey and Manning conclude:

> "How are we different from all the rest of life? The paleoanthropologist Ian Tattersall offers a good summary. 'To put this at its most elementary, humans care at least to some extent about each other's welfare; and chimpanzees as well as probably all of our other primate relatives do not. Our other primate relatives (Neanderthals etc.) did not—at least not to the extent we do—and they are extinct.'"[234]

If the defining characteristic of human society is caring, then we say that the crucial foundation this characteristic rests on is a loving, monogamous relationship. Monogamy makes family possible and workable. Family, in turn, makes a caring and cooperative human society not only possible, but probable. And interestingly enough, just as in Dr. Mlodinow's positive illusions research, one of the key factors that leads to lifelong romance is positive illusions. In a meta-analysis of 470 studies on marital compatibility, Dr. Marcel Zentner found that men and women who continue to believe that their spouse is attractive, funny, kind, and the ideal mate for them in almost every way remain content with each other. Social neuroscientist Dr. Bianca Acevedo, who is an expert in romantic love, agrees and says that one of the most important things linked with sustaining love over time is thinking positive things about your spouse. She says a key is for people to be able to let go of minor wrongs. See the best in your partner and look for humor. She recommends celebrating one another in large and small ways and not being apologetic about being crazy about your spouse even after many years.[235] The kind of positive mental attitude that has helped us survive and achieve great things in the past can also help us achieve great and lasting marriages.

This is why we feel so strongly about the importance of the insights shared in *Battles of the Sexes* to young adults.

We Are Survivors

It turns out that not only does the success of our species depend on our oxytocin-based caring and cooperation, but so does our very survival. And this, we argue, is highly dependent on our monogamous fidelity, which is the cornerstone for solid families. This is why, despite the challenges, we believe that loving and monogamous relationships that may go against our more polygynous nature are well worth it. The human condition, particularly when it comes to the Battles of the Sexes, has had a very complex developmental period. As Dr. Sarah Blaffer Hrdy puts it:

"Throughout much of evolutionary history, the uncertainty of paternity has been one of the several advantages females retained in a game otherwise heavily weighted towards male muscle mass. Female primates evolved a variety of strategies to pursue this advantage—the shift to situation dependent receptivity, concealed ovulation, and assertive sexuality. Such attributes improved the ability of females to manipulate males and to elicit from them the care and tolerance needed to rear the infants they bore. Females were abetted in this by selection by males themselves to promote the survival of infants which were likely, or even just possibly, their own."[236]

All of these factors may combine with what Paul Zak found with testosterone in men over their lifespan. The average age of becoming a father in the US is 29 years old. Testosterone starts to decline naturally around age 30, which helps men become less aggressive and have higher levels of empathy as they age. At the same time, the prefrontal cortex finally matures in men, which allows our rational executive functioning brain to better govern impulsivity, which leads to more controlled, rational thinking. As pointed out earlier, if a man commits to a woman, testosterone also declines, and if children are a result of this union, then testosterone levels go down even more. Both the factors that are at work in females and males bring hope to the prospect of establishing life-long monogamy. The most potent though, in these Battles of the Sexes, is as David Barash says: "Gaining an understanding of the predispositions that our ancestral history has made an integral part of us."

It is in this way that we can be most free from their magnetic pull. We can have the strength of will and self-mastery to go against their grain.

"Let's be clear: monogamy isn't natural, but as emphasized in the previous chapters, some of the best things we do aren't those that come naturally, but that involve hard work, often going specifically against our inclinations. It is easier to be lazy than to do good work, easier not to learn a second language, not to practice playing the violin, to be a couch potato instead of an athlete. It is easy to do what comes naturally: to breathe when our CO_2 levels reach a certain level, to sleep when tired, eat when hungry, drink when thirsty, and yes, have sex when horny. None of these things, however, are uniquely human. All are deeply biological and none especially admirable. To be maximally useful, 'Sex Ed' should therefore go beyond merely the birds and the bees, and details of male-female plumbing; it needs to educate people about their own sexual nature, which includes preparation for the pull of polygamy."

Dr. Barash points out that even though monogamy may not be natural for humans, there are biological mechanisms that can make it possible. One is the natural tendency for humans to attach themselves to other humans. This pattern begins right after birth as a baby will attach itself to its parents. It continues with most people as they form attachments to others throughout their lives. Sometimes this attachment inclination can lead to the greatest attachment of all: a loving marriage.

Another human biological characteristic that may support marriage is brain neuroplasticity. Neurons are constantly changed, molded, and improved through experience. This means that being around someone a great deal can help mold the two people's brains to synchronize more and more as years go by. That's how some couples' mannerisms become so similar over time.

Mirror neurons are another biological mechanism that may help marriages survive and even flourish. These brain cells allow us to actually vicariously feel what another is going through. Some neuroscientists call these empathy neurons. Dr. Barash asked whether they could also be called attachment neurons, bonding neurons, or even monogamy neurons?

We think there is a good possibility that this is the case.

Finally, Dr. Barash refers to Dr. Zak's favorite hormone— oxytocin—as being a possible factor in supporting happy, lifelong marriages. He cites the evidence from the prairie voles research that shows how important it is to the female's monogamous bonding.[237] From Dr. Zak's studies, it is obvious that oxytocin plays a major role in human relationships. We believe that it also plays a major role in permanent human pair-bonding.

Taken all together, we agree that these recently discovered biological factors lend themselves to raising the probability of successful marriages. Again, as Dr. Barash said, it is not natural though for many humans, and especially many human males. All of the elements that are part of human sexual nature are numerous and complex. We concur with Dr. Barash, who believes that the best chance for a young adult to successfully navigate these turbulent relational waters is to have a good understanding of their sexual nature, thus the IQ element of SEX IQ.

Simply Put

Einstein urged us to simplify as much as possible. In summary, we believe there are three major battles that young adults in the twenty-first century must face because of the mismatch we now have between our genetically-encoded sexual nature and our vastly changed modern culture. Using loose meanings for the operational words, for purposes of clarity, simplicity and understanding, and in view of the legacy of our polygynous past, here are the Major Battles of the Sexes:

1. Young men against their own sexual addictions
2. Young women against their own food addictions
3. Young women against young men's sex addictions

We believe these battles can, and should, be won.

And there is already one scientifically proven example of lasting romantic love. Dr. Helen Fisher worked with lead researcher Dr. Bianca Acevedo in 2007 to see if they could find examples of people who were still madly in love with their longtime spouse. Eventually, they found seventeen such people who were mostly in their fifties and had been married for an average of twenty-one years. They scanned their brains as these people looked at a picture of their spouse. Previously, psychologists believed that the dizzying feelings of romantic love lasted only about eighteen months or at most three years. Yet the brains of these midlife women and men showed very similar activity to brain scans of young lovers who had been intensely in love an average of only seven months. The only difference was that the older lovers' brain regions associated with anxiety were no longer active and instead there was increased activity in areas associated with calmness. It is important that we know that this can happen on its own. Dr. Acevedo's further research shows that for up to 40 percent of long-married couples, this lasting love may be the case.[238] We must remember though that this still leaves the majority of 60 percent who currently don't find lifelong wedded bliss. This would indicate the likely accuracy of Dr. Barash's assertion that monogamy is not natural for many humans, and we would add, especially for many human males.

Sexual Peace University

As Dr. Barash said, the key is a kind of 'New Sex Ed' that includes the unconscious motivating factors that come from our polygynous past. This new, more contextual approach to relationship education has also been advocated by Dr. Glenn Geher and Dr. Scott Barry Kaufman.[239] They too call for educating young people about the big picture of all of the different factors that are a part of sex and romantic love. They have even created an ingenious Mating Intelligence Scale that can be applied.

Additionally, the 2017 Harvard research project named "The Talk" showed that big numbers of young adults are presently unprepared for caring, lasting, romantic relationships and are nervous about developing them. It appears that parents and educators are not providing much guidance in these areas. The good news is that a large percentage of young people want this guidance. As a matter of fact, 65 percent of the thousands of 18-25 year olds surveyed wished they had received coaching on some aspect of romantic relationships in a health or sex education class in school. It is clear that these young people are open to, and even have a thirst for, knowledge about romantic love, which is very good because again it is projected that 85-90 percent of them will eventually marry. College may be the last formalized chance for education on young adult's sexuality. Most sex education the study reported presently is either focused narrowly on abstinence or is a disaster prevention approach aimed at preventing pregnancy and sexually transmitted infections.

The research team recommended that parents and educators talk about love and help young adults understand the differences between mature love and other forms of intense attraction. They advise teaching how to develop love and healthy relationships by exploring the differences between infatuation, intoxication, and love. The young adults can be asked to identify examples of healthy and unhealthy relationships in their own lives and in the media. One set of characteristics of a healthy romantic relationship is whether it makes both partners more respectful, compassionate, and hopeful. This relational education of young adults can go beyond romantic relationships and also cover what it means to act ethically overall and treat others of similar and different genders and races with caring and respect.

Dr. Rick Weissbourd, Faculty Director of Human Development and Psychology at Harvard, very aptly stated, "We spend an enormous amount of attention helping parents prepare their kids for work and school. We do almost nothing to prepare them for the tender, tough, subtle, generous, focused work of developing mature healthy relationships. I'm troubled by that. It may be the most important thing we do in life: learn how to love and be loved"[240]

We couldn't be more in agreement, and along those same lines, we propose a new healthy relationship educational program. We call it SEX IQ, and its mission is to bring these understandings to the young adult demographic at large. Research has already established that more intelligent males value monogamy. Data from a large representative US sample shows that boys who score higher on intelligence tests are more likely to grow up to value monogamy than their less intelligent male friends as they enter young adulthood.[241] We believe this monogamy intellect can be enhanced through our SEX IQ program for young adults. This book and its resulting program are dedicated to making a positive difference in young adults' lives. In this way, not only can couples live happily ever after, but can also benefit our human society as a whole.

You may be asking how promotion of lifelong romantic love can have benefits that go beyond the particular couple and ripple throughout our entire society.

Like we mentioned earlier, romantically pair-bonded couples are the cornerstones of families worldwide and Dr. James Heckman, a Nobel Prize winning economist from the University of Chicago, has shown through his research how strengthening families can positively affect the future. In a landmark paper written in 2011, Dr. Heckman stated that a key factor in determining a child's future success is whether he or she grows up in a one or two parent family.[242] There are many potential ingredients of lifetime success enmeshed in this one important variable in the human condition.

Obviously, there has been a great amount of change in our Western societies technologically and otherwise over the years. This has exacerbated the mismatchs we have described throughout *Battles of the Sexes*. We believe that this program, in combination with educational and other institutions, can make an even bigger positive difference in this repairable long-term relationship challenge. As we now know, a key weapon in this battle is education—understanding our human sexual nature.

The mismatch between the conditions and expectations of our ancestors' society and our present society can feel like a prison sentence, and sometimes actually lead to a literal prison sentence for behaviors that were naturally acted upon and carried out in the past.

We believe that the insights of *Battles of the Sexes* can help young adults understand and learn to constructively control their sexual nature. Our hope is that by knowing the truth, the truth shall make you free.

—— A SARAH SUMMARY: ——

- Monogamy can be difficult, but it is possible to achieve and serves the greater good of humanity. Just as you must have education, diligence, and willpower to learn an instrument, we as humans in the twenty-first century need the same for the upkeep of healthy, committed relationships with the opposite sex.
- Maintain variety and find adventure and enjoyment in relationships and develop a persistent intentionality to protect the union.
- Practice sexual transmutation: take control of sexual energy and focus it positively in other areas when giving in to the temptation could be ruinous to yourself or others.
- Men can win the battle against their sexual addictions; women can win the battle against their food addictions and against the sexually addictive tendencies of men.

Calling for a New Sex Ed

• • • • • • • • • • • • • • • • • • • •

"Those who don't know the past are doomed to repeat it"
EDMUND BURKE

We have one last bit of 'food for thought', if you will.

What do all of these people have in common?

Bill Clinton - 1998

Chris Matthews – 1999

Arnold Schwarzenegger – 2004

Mark Sanford – 2009

Tiger Woods – 2009

Anthony Weiner – 2011

Dominique Strass-Kahn – 2011

Bill Cosby - 2014

Donald Trump – 2016

Harvey Weinstein, Matt Lauer, Dustin Hoffman and many more – 2017

Andrew Creighton, Michael Douglas, Scott Baio - 2018

? – 2019

? – 2020

? – 2021

? – 2022
? – 2023, 2024, 2025...

That's right. The one thing they have in common is that they are high profile human males who have been accused of some kind of sexual misconduct. These are just the famous ones. Think how many more incidents occur that never make headlines! The male tendency to be sexually aggressive crosses all political party lines, nationalities, racial lines, socio-economic levels, and even age. It is an equal opportunity destroyer, especially for men, because of some high-testosterone males' inclination for reckless decision making.

Can that tendency really be due to socialization alone?

Or could there be biological forces involved that make greater sexual aggression a common trait for men worldwide? If so, perhaps the most effective way to combat it and prevent it is to understand the biochemistry and anatomy creating its motivational forces.

The methods used to draw attention to and fight this phenomenon have obviously not worked so far. Laws and corporate rules against sexual misconduct have been on the books for decades now. Do we really think we can solve this challenge through more rules alone?

> *"Insanity is doing the same thing over and over again and expecting different results"*
> ALBERT EINSTEIN

We believe it is time to employ all available knowledge, **including** natural, science-based knowledge to combat this regrettable situation and to indeed live romantically ever after.

In 2025, the 100th anniversary of the Scopes Trial (Dayton TN) will be observed. Will the lessons learned from scientific research on natural and sexual selection be applied to our challenges in the area of sexual conflict? Will we use this knowledge to raise SEX IQ and lower sexual conflict?

We certainly hope so.

"Lust is a Reaction. Love is a Decision"
Dr. Joe Malone

Thank You

• • • • • • • •

Thank you, dear reader, for reading this far. Without your support, none of this would be possible.

For updated news content related to Battles of the Sexes and information on the accompanying educational speaking program, SEX IQ, please visit sexiq.org or our SEX IQ facebook page at: https://www.facebook.com/SEX-IQ-1774364566199633/

About the Authors

· · · · · · · · · · · · · ·

Joe Malone holds a Ph.D. in Health and Human Performance with a minor in neuropsychology and a specialization in relational wellness. He has taught for many years at Middle Tennessee State University and guest lectured at Vanderbilt University. Dr. Malone served on the Centers for Disease Control Initiative for STD Prevention for the state of Tennessee. He has had 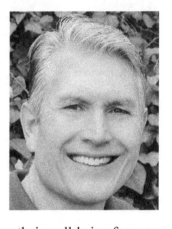 the honor of working with young adults on their well-being for over 25 years. In his teaching, Dr. Malone has employed a background of varied life experiences which include Division I football coach and player, fitness professional, and celebrity trainer as well as professional modeling. He has personally made use of the research, insights, and experience that inspired *Battles of the Sexes* and has had his SEX IQ raised to improve, preserve, and protect his over-40-year marriage to his wife, Jody. Dr. Malone and Jody make their home near their children and grandchildren in Nashville, TN.

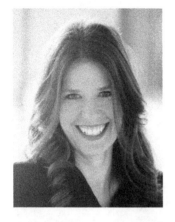

Sarah Harris is a graduated student of Dr. Malone who offers fresh perspective as a young adult herself, navigating many of the battles of culture versus nature that the female gender faces during reproductive years. She offers expertise in nutrition as a Registered Dietitian with over 5 years of experience providing nutrition counseling, and shares practical and realistic diet strategies to maintain optimal physical health. Sarah resides with her husband Scott and their children in Nashville, TN.

Notes

• • • • •

Introduction

1.   Trofimova, Irina. "A study of the dynamics of sex differences in adulthood". *International Journal of Psychology, 2013.*

2.   Geary David. *Male, Female: The Evolution of Human Sex Differences.* Washington, D.C.: American Psychological Association, 2010.

3.   Henig, Robin Marantz., and Samantha Henig. *Twentysomething: Why Do Young Adults Seem Stuck?* NY, NY: Plume, 2013.

4.   Jay, Meg. *The Defining Decade: Why Your Twenties Matter and How to Make the Most of Them Now.* Edinburgh: Canongate, 2016.

5.   Thornburg, Kent. *A Very Brief Description of Developmental Origins of Health and Disease.* Oregon Health & Science University, 2011.

Chapter 1

6.   Ratey, John J., Richard Manning, and David Perlmutter. *Go Wild: Eat Fat, Run Free, Be Social, and Follow Evolution's Other Rules for Total Health and Well-being.* New York, NY: Little, Brown, 2015.

7.   "Global Burden of Disease." *Lancet, 2012.*

8.   Ratey, John J., Richard Manning, and David Perlmutter. *Go Wild: Eat Fat, Run Free, Be Social, and Follow Evolution's Other Rules*

for Total Health and Well-being. New York, NY: Little, Brown, 2015.

9. "Behavioral Risk Factor Surveillance System." *Centers for Disease Control and Prevention*. August 29, 2017. Accessed October 09, 2017. https://www.cdc.gov/brfss/data_documentation/index.htm.

10. Lenhart, Amanda. *Teens, Smartphones & Texting*. (Washington D.C.:Pew Internet and American Life Project, 2012).

11. Pinker, Susan. *The Village Effect: How Face-to-face Contact Can Make Us Healthier and Happier.* Toronto: Vintage Canada, 2015.

12. Ibid.

13. Preisler, Andy. "Recent Research Finds Millennials Are the Best Educated Yet Worst Paid Generation."

14. Ibid.

15. Ibid.

16. Trofimova, Irina. "A study of the dynamics of sex differences in adulthood". *International Journal of Psychology*, 2013.

17. Epstein, David J. *The Sports Gene: What Makes the Perfect Athlete.* Rearsby, Leicester: WF Howes, 2013.

18. Ibid.

19. Pinker, Steven. *The Blank Slate: The Modern Denial of Human Nature.* London: Penguin, 2003.

20. Cross, Catharine P., Lee T. Copping, and Anne Campbell. "Sex Differences in Impulsivity: A Meta-analysis." *Psychological Bulletin* 137, no. 1 (2011): 97-130. doi:10.1037/a0021591.

21. Rommelse., Nanda. "Relationship between Endophenotype and Phenotype in ADHD." *Behavioral Brain Function*, 2008.

22. Geary David. Male, Female: *The Evolution of Human Sex Differences.* Washington, D.C.: American Psychological Association, 2010.

23. Ibid.

24. Hamann, Stephan. "Men and Women Differ in Amygdala Response to Visual Sexual Stimuli." 2004. doi:10.1038/nn1208.

25. Zak, Paul J. *Moral Molecule: How Trust Works*. NY, NY: Penguin Group, 2013.

26. Wang, Gene-Jack, et al. "Evidence of gender differences in the ability to inhibit brain activation elicited by food stimulation". *Proceedings of the National Academy of Science* 106(4):1249-54. (2009). doi: 10.1073/pnas.0807423106.

27. "Behavioral Risk Factor Surveillance System." *Centers for Disease Control and Prevention*. August 29, 2017. Accessed October 09, 2017.

28. Ferrara, Cynthia. "The college experience: physical activity, nutrition, and implications for intervention and future research." *Journal of Online Physiology*, 2009.

29. Han, Jennifer, et al. "Changes in women's physical activity during the transition to college".*American Journal of Health Education*, 39 (4), 2008.

30. Lassek, William D., and Steven J. C. Gaulin. *Why Women Need Fat: How "healthy" Food Makes Us Gain Excess Weight and the Surprising Solution to Losing It Forever*. New York: Hudson Street Press, 2012.

31. Flegal, Katherine M. "Trends in Obesity Among Adults in the United States, 2005 to 2014." *JAMA*. June 07, 2016. Accessed October 09, 2017. http://jamanetwork.com/journals/jama/fullarticle/2526639.

32. Gluckman, Peter D., and Mark A. Hanson. Mismatch: *The Lifestyle Diseases Timebomb*. Oxford: Oxford University Press, 2013.

Chapter 2

33. Trevathan, Wenda. *Ancient Bodies, Modern Lives: How Evolution Has Shaped Women's Health.* New York: Oxford University Press, 2010.

34. Short, Roger. "The evolution of human reproduction." *Proceedings of the Royal Society of London* Series B –Biological Sciences 195: 3-24.

35. Trevathan, Wenda. Ancient Bodies, *Modern Lives: How Evolution Has Shaped Women's Health*. New York: Oxford University Press, 2010.

36. Rankin, Lissa. *What's up down There?* London: Robert Hale, 2010.

37. Tietze, C. Reproductive span and rate of reproduction among Hutterite women. *Fertility and Sterility*, 1957.

38. Lichterman, Gabrielle. *28 Days*. Avon, MA: Adams Media, 2005.

39. Smolensky, Michael H., and Lynne Lamberg. *The Body Clock Guide to Better Health: How to Use Your Body's Natural Clock to Fight Illness and Achieve Maximum Health.* New York: H. Holt, 2001.

40. Lichterman, Gabrielle. *28 Days*. Avon, MA: Adams Media, 2005.

41. Smolensky, Michael H., and Lynne Lamberg. *The Body Clock Guide to Better Health: How to Use Your Body's Natural Clock to Fight Illness and Achieve Maximum Health*. New York: H. Holt, 2001.

42. Perrett, DI. "Menstrual cycle alters face preference." 1996.

43. Cowley, Geoffrey. *The Biology of Beauty.*1996.

44. Bellis, Mark A., and R. Robin Baker. "Do Females Promote Sperm Competition? Data for Humans." *Sperm Competition in Humans*: 135-39. doi:10.1007/0-387-28039-1_9.

45. Lichterman, Gabrielle. 28 Days. Avon, MA: Adams Media, 2005.

Chapter 3

46. Wang, Gene-Jack, et al. "Evidence of gender differences in the ability to inhibit brain activation elicited by food stimulation". *Proceedings of the National Academy of Science* 106(4):1249-54. (2009). doi: 10.1073/pnas.0807423106.

47. Hamann. "Men and Women Differ in Amygdala Response to Visual Sexual Stimuli." 2004. doi:10.1038/nn1208.

48. Lieberman, Daniel. *The Story of the Human Body: Evolution, Health, and Disease. New York: Vintage Books, 2014.*

49. *Geary David. Male, Female: The Evolution of Human Sex Differences.* Washington, D.C.: American Psychological Association, 2010.

50. Wurtman, Judith J., and Susan Suffes. *The Serotonin Solution.* New York: Fawcett Columbine, 1997.

51. Lassek, William D., and Steven J. C. Gaulin. *Why Women Need Fat: How "healthy" Food Makes Us Gain Excess Weight and the Surprising Solution to Losing It Forever.* New York: Hudson Street Press, 2012.

52. Thornburg, Kent. *A Very Brief Description of Developmental Origins of Health and Disease.* Oregon Health & Science University, 2011.

Chapter 4

53. Brizendine, Louann. *The Male Brain.* New York: Three Rivers Press, 2010.

54. Roach, Mary. *Bonk: The Curious Coupling of Science and Sex.* New York: W.W. Norton &, 2009.

55. Howard, Pierce. *The Owner's Manual for the Brain.* New York: Harper Collins, 2014.

56. Baker, Jennifer. Forest Institute of Professional Psychiatry

57. Howard, Pierce. *The Owner's Manual for the Brain.* New York: Harper Collins, 2014.

58. Barash, David P. *Out of Eden the Surprising Consequences of Polygamy.* New York: Oxford University Press, 2016.

59. Wilson, M., and M. Daly. "Do Pretty Women Inspire Men to Discount the Future?" *Proceedings of the Royal Society B*: Biological Sciences 271, no. Suppl_4 (2004). doi:10.1098/rsbl.2003.0134.

60. Ariely, Dan, and George Loewenstein. "The Heat of the Moment: The Effect of Sexual Arousal on Sexual Decision Making." *Journal of Behavioral Decision Making* 19, no. 2 (2006): 87-98. doi:10.1002/bdm.501.

61. Karren, Keith: Hafen: Brent: Smith, Lee: Frandsen, Kathryn. *Mind body health: The effects of attitudes, emotions and relationships.* San Francisco: Pearson Benjamin Cummings, 2006.

62. Zak, Paul J. Moral Molecule: How Trust Works. NY, NY: Penguin Group, 2013.

63. Bondar, Carin. *Wild Sex: The Science behind Mating in the Animal Kingdom.* New York: Pegasus Books, 2016.

Chapter 5

64. Medina, John. *The Genetic Inferno: Inside the Seven Deadly Sins. Cambridge:* Cambridge University Press, 2012.

65. Miller, Geoffrey, Joshua M. Tybur, and Brent D. Jordan. "Ovulatory Cycle Effects on Tip Earnings by Lap Dancers: Economic Evidence for Human Estrus?â˜†." *Evolution and Human Behavior* 28, no. 6 (2007): 375-81. doi:10.1016/j.evolhumbehav.2007.06.002.

66. Singh, D., and P. M. Bronstad. "Female Body Odour Is a Potential Cue to Ovulation." *Proceedings of the Royal Society B: Biological Sciences* 268, no. 1469 (2001): 797-801. doi:10.1098/rspb.2001.1589.

67. Pincott, J. *Do Gentlemen Really Prefer Blondes?: Why He Fancies You and Why He Doesn't.* London: Bantam Press, 2008.

68. Thornhill, R. "The Scent of Symmetry A Human Sex Pheromone That Signals Fitness?" *Evolution and Human Behavior* 20, no. 3 (1999): 175-201. doi:10.1016/s1090-5138(99)00005-7.

69. Pincott, J. *Do Gentlemen Really Prefer Blondes?: Why He Fancies You and Why He Doesn't.* London: Bantam Press, 2008.

70. Smith, M.j Law, D.i Perrett, B.c Jones, R.e Cornwell, F.r Moore, D.r Feinberg, L.g Boothroyd, S.j Durrani, M.r Stirrat, S. Whiten, R.m Pitman, and S.g Hillier. "Facial Appearance Is a Cue to Oestrogen Levels in Women." *Proceedings of the Royal Society B*: Biological Sciences 273, no. 1583 (2006): 135-40. doi:10.1098/rspb.2005.3296.

71. Lichterman, Gabrielle. *28 Days.* Avon, MA: Adams Media, 2005.

72. Durante, Kristina M., Norman P. Li, and Martie G. Haselton. "Changes in Women's Choice of Dress Across the Ovulatory Cycle: Naturalistic and Laboratory Task-Based Evidence." *Personality and Social Psychology Bulletin* 34, no. 11 (2008): 1451-460. doi:10.1177/0146167208323103.

73. Chavanne, Tara J., and Gordon G. Gallup. "Variation in Risk Taking Behavior Among Female College Students as a Function of the Menstrual Cycle." Evolution and Human Behavior 19, no. 1 (1998): 27-32. doi:10.1016/s1090-5138(98)00016-6.

74. "Supplemental Material for Do Womens Mate Preferences Change Across the Ovulatory Cycle? A Meta-Analytic Review." *Psychological Bulletin*, 2014. doi:10.1037/a0035438.supp.

75. Baker, Robin. Bellis, Mark. *Human sperm competition: Copulation, masturbation and infidelity.* New New York: Springer, 1994.

76. Howard, Pierce. *The Owner's Manual for the Brain.* New York: Harper Collins, 2014.

Chapter 6

77. Young, Larry, and Brian Alexander. *The Chemistry between Us: Love, Sex, and the Science of Attraction.* New York: Current, 2012.

78. Lassek, William D., and Steven J. C. Gaulin. *Why Women Need Fat: How "healthy" Food Makes Us Gain Excess Weight and the Surprising Solution to Losing It Forever.* New York: Hudson Street Press, 2012.

79. Buss, David M. *The Evolution of Desire: Strategies of Human Mating.* New York: Basic Books, 2016.

80. Lassek, William D., and Steven J. C. Gaulin. *Why Women Need Fat: How "healthy" Food Makes Us Gain Excess Weight and the Surprising Solution to Losing It Forever.* New York: Hudson Street Press, 2012.

81. Bainbridge, David. Curvology: *The Origins and Power of Female Body Shape.* New York: Overlook Press, 2016.

82. Lassek, William D., and Steven J. C. Gaulin. *Why Women Need Fat: How "healthy" Food Makes Us Gain Excess Weight and the Surprising Solution to Losing It Forever.* New York: Hudson Street Press, 2012.

83. Lieberman, Daniel. *The Story of the Human Body: Evolution, Health, and Disease.* New York: Vintage Books, 2014.

84. Lassek, William D., and Steven J. C. Gaulin. *Why Women Need Fat: How "healthy" Food Makes Us Gain Excess Weight and the Surprising Solution to Losing It Forever.* New York: Hudson Street Press, 2012.

85. Geary David. *Male, Female: The Evolution of Human Sex Differences*. Washington, D.C. American Psychological Association, 2010.

Chapter 7

86. Buss, David M. *The Evolution of Desire: Strategies of Human Mating.* New York: Basic Books, 2016.

87. Kanazawa, Satoshi. Why More Intelligent Men (But Not Women) Value Sexual Exclusivity. *Psychology Today* Online, April 19, 2010.

88. Buss, David M. *The Evolution of Desire: Strategies of Human Mating*. New York: Basic Books, 2016.

89. Zak, Paul J. *Moral Molecule: How Trust Works*. NY, NY: Penguin Group, 2013.

90. Ibid.

91. Hrdy, Sarah. *The Woman Who Never Evolved*. Cambridge: The President and Fellows of Harvard College, 1999.

92. Sherfey, Mary Jane. *The Nature and Evolution of Female Sexuality.* New York: Random House, 1973.

93. Herbenick, Debby, and Vanessa Schick. *Read My Lips: A Complete Guide to the Vagina and Vulva.* Lanham: Rowman & Littlefield Publishers, 2011.

94. Sherfey, Mary Jane. *The Nature and Evolution of Female Sexuality*. New York: Random House, 1973.

95. Haller, Katie. *"The Truth behind Why Women Find It Harder to Have Casual Sex than Men Do."* 2014.

96. Pincott, J. *Do Gentlemen Really Prefer Blondes?: Why He Fancies You and Why He Doesn't.* London: Bantam Press, 2008.

97. Fielder, Robyn L., and Michael P. Carey. "Predictors and Consequences of Sexual Hookups Among College Students: A

Short-term Prospective Study." *Archives of Sexual Behavior* 39, no. 5 (2009): 1105-119. doi:10.1007/s10508-008-9448-4.

Chapter 8

98. Buss, David M. *The Evolution of Desire: Strategies of Human Mating.* New York: Basic Books, 2016.

99. Saxon, Lynn. *Sex at Dusk: Lifting the Shiny Wrapping from Sex at Dawn.* Leipzig: Amazon, 2012.

100. Birkhead, T. R. "Defining And Demonstrating Postcopulatory Female Choice Again." *Evolution* 54, no. 3 (2000): 1057. doi:10.1554/0014-3820(2000)054[1057:dadpfc]2.3.co;2.

101. Gorelik, Gregory, and Todd K. Shackelford. "Human Sexual Conflict from Molecules to Culture." *Evolutionary Psychology* 9, no. 4 (2011): 147470491100900. doi:10.1177/147470491100900408.

102. Jr., Gordon G. Gallup, Rebecca L. Burch, and Steven M. Platek. *Archives of Sexual Behavior* 31, no. 3 (2002): 289-93. doi:10.1023/a:1015257004839.

103. Gottschall, Jonathan A., and Tiffani A. Gottschall. "Are Per-incident Rape-pregnancy Rates Higher than Per-incident Consensual Pregnancy Rates?" *SpringerLink.* Accessed October 02, 2017. https://link.springer.com/article/10.1007/s12110-003-1014-0.

104. Robin Baker and Mark A. Bellis. "Human Sperm Competition: Ejaculate Manipulation by Females and a Function for the Female Orgasm (1993)." *Sperm Competition in Humans*: 177-210. doi:10.1007/978-0-387-28039-4_11.

105. Chartrand, Tanya L. and John A. Bargh. *"The Chameleon Effect: The Perception-behavior Link and Social Interaction."* Journal of Personality and Social Psychology 76, no. 6 (1999): 893-910. doi:10.1037//0022-3514.76.6.893.

106. Paul, Jr. Costa, Antonio Terracciano, and Robert R. Mccrae. "Gender Differences in Personality Traits across Cultures: Robust and Surprising Findings." *Journal of Personality and Social Psychology* 81, no. 2 (2001): 322-31. doi:10.1037//0022-3514.81.2.322.

107. Kruger, Daniel J., and Randolph M. Nesse. "Sexual Selection and the Male:Female Mortality Ratio." *Evolutionary Psychology* 2, no. 1 (2004): 147470490400200. doi:10.1177/147470490400200112.

108. Cross, Catharine P., Lee T. Copping, and Anne Campbell. "Sex Differences in Impulsivity: A Meta-analysis." *Psychological Bulletin* 137, no. 1 (2011): 97-130. doi:10.1037/a0021591.

109. Struber, Daniel, Monika Luck, and Gerhard Roth. "Sex, Aggression and Impulse Control: An Integrative Account." *Neurocase* 14, no. 1 (2008): 93-121. doi:10.1080/13554790801992743.

110. Archer, John. "Sex Differences in Aggression in Real-World Settings: A Meta-Analytic Review." *Review of General Psychology* 8, no. 4 (2004): 291-322. doi:10.1037/1089-2680.8.4.291.

111. "Idaho State Department of Education (SDE)." SDE. Accessed October 03, 2017. https://www.sde.idaho.gov/.

112. Bishop, Phillip, Kirk Cureton, and Mitchell Collins. "Sex Difference in Muscular Strength in Equally-trained Men and Women." *Ergonomics* 30, no. 4 (1987): 675-87. doi:10.1080/00140138708969760.

113. Halpern, Diane F. Sex Differences in Cognitive Abilities. New York: *Psychology Press*, 2012.

114. Ibid.

115. Baron-Cohen, Simon, Michael V. Lombardo, Bonnie Auyeung, Emma Ashwin, Bhismadev Chakrabarti, and Rebecca Knickmeyer. "Why Are Autism Spectrum Conditions More Prevalent in Males?" *PLoS Biology* 9, no. 6 (2011). doi:10.1371/journal.pbio.1001081.

116. Leaper, Campbell, and Rachael D. Robnett. "Women Are More Likely Than Men to Use Tentative Language, Aren't They? A Meta-Analysis Testing for Gender Differences and Moderators." *Psychology of Women Quarterly* 35, no. 1 (2011): 129-42. doi:10.1177/0361684310392728.

117. Trofimova, Irina. "An Investigation into Differences between the Structure of Temperament and the Structure of Personality." *The American Journal of Psychology* 123, no. 4 (2010): 467. doi:10.5406/amerjpsyc.123.4.0467.

118. Browne, Kingsley. *Biology at Work: Rethinking Sexual Equality.* New Brunswick, NJ: Rutgers University Press, 2002.

119. Cross, Catharine P., Lee T. Copping, and Anne Campbell. "Sex Differences in Impulsivity: A Meta-analysis." *Psychological Bulletin* 137, no. 1 (2011): 97-130. doi:10.1037/a0021591.

120. Baron-Cohen, Simon, Michael V. Lombardo, Bonnie Auyeung, Emma Ashwin, Bhismadev Chakrabarti, and Rebecca Knickmeyer. "Why Are Autism Spectrum Conditions More Prevalent in Males?" *PLoS Biology* 9, no. 6 (2011). doi:10.1371/journal.pbio.1001081.

121. Halpern, Diane F. *Sex Differences in Cognitive Abilities.* New York: Psychology Press, 2012.

122. Kuhle, Barry X. "It's Funny Because It's True (because It Evokes Our Evolved Psychology)." *Review of General Psychology* 16, no. 2 (2012): 177-86. doi:10.1037/a0027912.

123. Haselton, Martie G., and David M. Buss. "Error Management Theory: A New Perspective on Biases in Cross-sex Mind Reading." *Journal of Personality and Social Psychology* 78, no. 1 (2000): 81-91. doi:10.1037//0022-3514.78.1.81.

124. Todd K. Shackelford, Aaron T. Goetz, Faith E. Guta, and David P. Schmitt. "Mate Guarding and Frequent In-pair Copulation in Humans." *Human Nature* 17, no. 3 (2006): 239-52. doi:10.1007/s12110-006-1007-x.

125. Buss, David M., Todd K. Shackelford, Lee A. Kirkpatrick, Jae C. Choe, Hang K. Lim, Mariko Hasegawa, Toshikazu Hasegawa, and Kevin Bennett. "Jealousy and the Nature of Beliefs about Infidelity: Tests of Competing Hypotheses about Sex Differences in the United States, Korea, and Japan." *Personal Relationships* 6, no. 1 (1999): 125-50. doi:10.1111/j.1475-6811.1999.tb00215.x.

126. Miner, Emily J., Valerie G. Starratt, and Todd K. Shackelford. "It's Not All about Her: Men's Mate Value and Mate Retention." *Personality and Individual Differences* 47, no. 3 (2009): 214-18. doi:10.1016/j.paid.2009.03.002.

127. Buss, David M. *The Evolution of Desire: Strategies of Human Mating.* New York: Basic Books, 2016.

128. Ibid.

129. Malone,Joe. *Creating a College Womens Wellness Program: Innovation for Health Promotion.* PhD diss., MTSU, 2015.

130. Ibid.

131. Buss, David M. *The Evolution of Desire: Strategies of Human Mating.* New York: Basic Books, 2016.

132. Studd, Michael V., and Urs E. Gattiker. "The Evolutionary Psychology of Sexual Harassment in Organizations." *Ethology and Sociobiology* 12, no. 4 (1991): 249-90. doi:10.1016/0162-3095(91)90021-h.

133. Gutek, Barbara. *Sex and the Workplace: The Impact of Sexual Behavior and Harassment on Women, Men, and the Organization.* San Francisco: Jossey Bass, 1985.

134. Impett, Emily A., and Letitia Anne Peplau. "Why Some Women Consent to Unwanted Sex With a Dating Partner: Insights from Attachment Theory." *Psychology of Women Quarterly* 26, no. 4 (2002): 360-70. doi:10.1111/1471-6402.t01-1-00075.

135. Thornhill, Randy, and Nancy Wilmsen Thornhill. "Human Rape: An Evolutionary Analysis." *Ethology and Sociobiology* 4, no. 3 (1983): 137-73. doi:10.1016/0162-3095(83)90027-4.

136. Malamuth, Neil M. "Rape Proclivity Among Males." *Journal of Social Issues* 37, no. 4 (1981): 138-57. doi:10.1111/j.1540-4560.1981.tb01075.x.

137. Young, Robert K., and Del Thiessen. "The Texas Rape Scale." *Ethology and Sociobiology* 13, no. 1 (1992): 19-33. doi:10.1016/0162-3095(92)90004-n.

138. Sexual Assault Center of Nashville Statistics, 2017.

139. Vanderbilt Rape Case, New York Post Online, August 18th 2017.

140. Lalumiere, Martin. *The Causes of Rape: Understanding Individual Differences in Male Propensity for Sexual Aggression.* Washington, DC: APA.

141. Malone, Joe. *Creating a College Womens Wellness Program: Innovation for Health Promotion.* PhD diss., MTSU, 2015. Pg. 78.

142. Malone, Joe. Pilot Study on Differences in P.E. Class Perceptions Between Males and Females, 2015.

143. Gorelik, Gregory, and Todd K. Shackelford. "Human Sexual Conflict from Molecules to Culture." *Evolutionary Psychology* 9, no. 4 (2011): 14747049110090doi:10.1177/147470491100900408.

Chapter 9

144. Malone, Joe. *Creating a College Womens Wellness Program: Innovation for Health Promotion.* PhD diss., MTSU, 2015.

145. Annis, Barbara and Merron, Keith. *Gender Intelligence: Breakthrough Strategies for Increasing Diversity and Improving Your Bottom Line.* New York: Harper Collins Publishers, 2014.

146. Fisher, Helen. *The First Sex: The Natural Talents of Women and How They Are Changing the World.* New York: Ballantine Books, 2000.

147. Annis, Barbara and Merron, Keith. *Gender Intelligence: Breakthrough Strategies for Increasing Diversity and Improving Your Bottom Line.* New York: Harper Collins Publishers, 2014.

148. Zak, Paul J. *Moral Molecule: How Trust Works.* NY, NY: Penguin Group, 2013.

149. Buss, David M. *The Evolution of Desire: Strategies of Human Mating.* New York: Basic Books, 2016.

Chapter 10

150. Hinshaw, Stephen P., and Rachel Kranz. *The Triple Bind: Saving Our Teenage Girls from Today's Pressures and Conflicting Expectations.* New York: Ballantine Books Trade Paperbacks, 2009.

151. Dennerlein, Liz. "Study: Females Lose Self-confidence throughout College." USA Today. September 26, 2013. Accessed September 28, 2017. https://www.usatoday.com/story/news/nation/2013/09/26/study-females-lose-confidence-college/2871111/.

152. "Spring 2013 National College Health Assessment."

153. "The American Freshman National Norms 2010"

154. Garcia, Justin R., Chris Reiber, Sean G. Massey, and Ann M. Merriwether. "Sexual Hook-up Culture." *PsycEXTRA* Dataset. doi:10.1037/e505012013-009.

155. Bogle. "The Shift from Dating to Hooking up in College What Scholars Have Missed." *Sociology Compass*, 2007.

156. Garcia, Justin R., Chris Reiber, Sean G. Massey, and Ann M. Merriwether. "Sexual Hook-up Culture." *PsycEXTRA* Dataset. doi:10.1037/e505012013-009.

157. Bogle. "The Shift from Dating to Hooking up in College What Scholars Have Missed." *Sociology Compass*, 2007.

158. Kunkel, D., Eyal, K., Finnerty, K., Biely, E., & Donnerstein, E. (2005). *Sex on TV 4: A biennial report to the Kaiser Family Foundation*. Menlo Park, CA: Kaiser Family Foundation.

159. Garcia, Justin R., Chris Reiber, Sean G. Massey, and Ann M. Merriwether. "Sexual Hook-up Culture." *PsycEXTRA* Dataset. doi:10.1037/e505012013-009.

160. Owen, Jesse, Frank D. Fincham, and Jon Moore. "Short-Term Prospective Study of Hooking Up Among College Students." *Archives of Sexual Behavior* 40, no. 2 (2011): 331-41. doi:10.1007/s10508-010-9697-x.

161. Paul, Elizabeth L., and Kristen A. Hayes. "The Casualties of 'Casual' Sex: A Qualitative Exploration of the Phenomenology of College Students' Hookups." *Journal of Social and Personal Relationships* 19, no. 5 (2002): 639-61. doi:10.1177/0265407502195006.

162. Ibid.

163. Pincott, J. *Do Gentlemen Really Prefer Blondes?: Why He Fancies You and Why He Doesn't*. London: Bantam Press, 2008.

164. Ariely, Dan, and George Loewenstein. "The Heat of the Moment: The Effect of Sexual Arousal on Sexual Decision Making." *Journal of Behavioral Decision Making* 19, no. 2 (2006): 87-98. doi:10.1002/bdm.501.

165. Lewis, Melissa A., Hollie Granato, Jessica A. Blayney, Ty W. Lostutter, and Jason R. Kilmer. "Predictors of Hooking Up Sexual Behaviors and Emotional Reactions Among U.S. College Students." SpringerLink. July 28, 2011. Accessed September 29, 2017. https://link.springer.com/article/10.1007/s10508-011-9817-2.

166. Oswalt, Sara B., Kenzie A. Cameron, and Jeffrey J. Koob. "Sexual Regret in College Students." *Archives of Sexual Behavior* 34, no. 6 (2005): 663-69. doi:10.1007/s10508-005-7920-y.

167. Eshbaugh, Elaine M., and Gary Gute. "Hookups and Sexual Regret Among College Women." *The Journal of Social Psychology* 148, no. 1 (2008): 77-90. doi:10.3200/socp.148.1.77-90.

168. Grello, Catherine M., Deborah P. Welsh, and Melinda S. Harper. "No Strings Attached: The Nature of Casual Sex in College Students." *Journal of Sex Research* 43, no. 3 (2006): 255-67. doi:10.1080/00224490609552324.

169. Lambert, Tracy A., Arnold S. Kahn, and Kevin J. Apple. "Pluralistic Ignorance and Hooking up." *Journal of Sex Research* 40, no. 2 (2003): 129-33. doi:10.1080/00224490309552174.

170. Reiber, Chris, and Justin R. Garcia. "Hooking Up: Gender Differences, Evolution, and Pluralistic Ignorance." *Evolutionary Psychology* 8, no. 3 (2010): 147470491000800. doi:10.1177/147470491000800307.

171. Herold, Edward S., and Dawn Arie K. Mewhinney. "Gender Differences in Casual Sex and AIDS Prevention: A Survey of Dating Bars." *Journal of Sex Research* 30, no. 1 (1993): 36-42. doi:10.1080/00224499309551676.

172. Garcia, Justin R., and Chris Reiber. "Hook-up Behavior: A Biopsychosocial Perspective." *Journal of Social, Evolutionary, and Cultural Psychology* 2, no. 4 (2008): 192-208. doi:10.1037/h0099345.

173. Garcia, Justin R., Chris Reiber, Sean G. Massey, and Ann M. Merriwether. "Sexual Hook-up Culture." *PsycEXTRA* Dataset. doi:10.1037/e505012013-009.

174. "Prevalence and Characteristics of Sexual Hookups among First-semester Female College Students." International Braz J Urol 36, no. 5 (2010): 643-44. doi:10.1590/s1677-55382010000500026. differences." *Archives of Sexual Behavior* 24, no. 2 (1995): 173-206. doi:10.1007/bf01541580.

175. Flack, William F., Kimberly A. Daubman, Marcia L. Caron, Jenica A. Asadorian, Nicole R. D'Aureli, Shannon N. Gigliotti, Anna T. Hall, Sarah Kiser, and Erin R. Stine. "Risk Factors and

Consequences of Unwanted Sex Among University Students." *Journal of Interpersonal Violence* 22, no. 2 (2007): 139-57. doi:10.1177/0886260506295354.

176. Freitas, Donna. *The End of Sex: How Hookup Culture Is Leaving a Generation Unhappy, Sexually Unfulfilled, and Confused about Intimacy*. New York: Basic Books, 2013.

177. Geher, Glenn, and Scott Barry Kaufman. *Mating Intelligence Unleashed: The Role of the Mind in Sex, Dating, and Love.* New York: Oxford University Press, 2013.

178. Samelson, Chelsea. "Are We Finally Unhooking from Hook Up Culture?" *Acculturated.* February 23, 2016. Accessed September 30, 2017. https://acculturated.com/unhooking-from-hook-up-culture/.

179. CDC Finds Sharp Growth in STDs in College-Age Population. Inside Higher Education Online, November 3, 2016.

180. McGuire, Ashley. *Sex Scandal: The Drive to Abolish Male and Female.* Washington, DC: Regnery Publishing, a Division of Salem Media Group, 2017.

181. Samelson, Chelsea. "Are We Finally Unhooking from Hook Up Culture?" *Acculturated.* February 23, 2016. Accessed September 30, 2017. https://acculturated.com/unhooking-from-hook-up-culture/.

182. "The Talk: How Adults Can Promote Young People's Healthy Relationships and Prevent Misogyny and Sexual Harassment." *Making Caring Common.* Accessed November 27, 2017. https://mcc.gse.harvard.edu/thetalk.

183. Oswalt, Sara B., Tammy J. Wyatt, and Yesenia Ochoa. "Sexual Assault Is Just the Tip of the Iceberg: Relationship and Sexual Violence Prevalence in College Students." *Journal of College Student Psychotherapy*, 2017, 1-17. doi:10.1080/87568225.2017.1350122.

184. Annis, Barbara and Merron, Keith. *Gender Intelligence: Breakthrough Strategies for Increasing Diversity and Improving Your Bottom Line.* New York: Harper Collins Publishers, 2014.

185. Brizendine, Louann. *The Female Brain.* London: Bantam, 2007.

186. Zaidi, Zeenat F. "Gender Differences in Human Brain: A Review." *The Open Anatomy Journal* 2 (2010): 37-55. doi:10.2174/18776094 01002010037.

187. Annis, Barbara and Merron, Keith. Gender *Intelligence: Breakthrough Strategies for Increasing Diversity and Improving Your Bottom Line.* New York: Harper Collins Publishers, 2014.

188. Blum, Deborah. *Sex on the Brain: The Biological Differences between Men and Women.* New York: Penguin, 1998.

189. Annis, Barbara and Merron, Keith. Gender *Intelligence: Breakthrough Strategies for Increasing Diversity and Improving Your Bottom Line.* New York: Harper Collins Publishers, 2014.

190. Cahill, Larry. *Equality Does Not Equal the Same.* Cerebrum, April, 2014.

191. Amen, Daniel. "Women Have More Active Brains Than Men." *Journal of Alzheimer's Disease* (2017).

192. Geary David. Male, Female: The Evolution of Human Sex Differences. Washington, D.C.: *American Psychological Association,* 2010.

193. Wilcox, Allen J., Clarice R. Weinberg, and Donna D. Baird. "Timing of Sexual Intercourse in Relation to Ovulation Effects on the Probability of Conception, Survival of the Pregnancy, and Sex of the Baby." *New England Journal of Medicine* 333, no. 23 (1995): 1517-521. doi:10.1056/nejm199512073332301.

194. Anders, Sari M. Van, Lisa Dawn Hamilton, and Neil V. Watson. "Multiple Partners Are Associated with Higher Testosterone in North American Men and Women." *Hormones and Behavior* 51, no. 3 (2007): 454-59. doi:10.1016/j.yhbeh.2007.01.002.

195. Gangestad, Steven W., and Randy Thornhill. "Human Oestrus." *Proceedings of the Royal Society of London B: Biological Sciences.* May 07, 2008. Accessed September 30, 2017. http://rspb. royalsocietypublishing.org/content/275/1638/991/.

196. Penton-Voak, Ian S., and David I. Perrett. "Male Facial Attractiveness: Perceived Personality and Shifting Female Preferences for Male Traits across the Menstrual Cycle." *Advances*

in the Study of Behavior, 2001, 219-59. doi:10.1016/s0065-3454(01)80008-5.

197. Slob, A. Koos, Cindy M. Bax, Wim C.j. Hop, David L. Rowland, and Jacob J. Van Der Werff Ten Bosch. "Sexual Arousability and the Menstrual Cycle." *Psychoneuroendocrinology* 21, no. 6 (1996): 545-58. doi:10.1016/0306-4530(95)00058-5.

198. "The Scent of Symmetry: A Human Sex Pheromone That Signals Fitness?" *Evolution and Human Behavior*. July 08, 1999. Accessed September 30, 2017. http://www.sciencedirect.com/science/article/pii/S1090513899000057.

199. Puts, David Andrew. "Mating Context and Menstrual Phase Affect Women's Preferences for Male Voice Pitch." *Evolution and Human Behavior* 26, no. 5 (2005): 388-97. doi:10.1016/j.evolhumbehav.2005.03.001. Geary David. Male, Female: The Evolution of Human Sex Differences. Washington, D.C.: American Psychological Association, 2010.

200. Haselton, Martie G., and Steven W. Gangestad. "Conditional Expression of Women's Desires and Men's Mate Guarding across the Ovulatory Cycle." *Hormones and Behavior* 49, no. 4 (2006): 509-18. doi:10.1016/j.yhbeh.2005.10.006.

201. Roney, James R., and Zachary L. Simmons. "Women's Estradiol Predicts Preference for Facial Cues of Men's Testosterone." *Hormones and Behavior* 53, no. 1 (2008): 14-19. doi:10.1016/j.yhbeh.2007.09.008.

202. Penton-Voak, Ian S., and David I. Perrett. "Male Facial Attractiveness: Perceived Personality and Shifting Female Preferences for Male Traits across the Menstrual Cycle." *Advances in the Study of Behavior*, 2001, 219-59. doi:10.1016/s0065-3454(01)80008-5.

203. Cherlin, Andrew J. "The Origins of the Ambivalent Acceptance of Divorce." *Journal of Marriage and Family* 71, no. 2 (2009): 226-29. doi:10.1111/j.1741-3737.2009.00593.x.

204. Easton, Judith A., Jaime C. Confer, Cari D. Goetz, and David M. Buss. "Reproduction Expediting: Sexual Motivations, Fantasies, and the Ticking Biological Clock." *Personality and*

Individual Differences 49, no. 5 (2010): 516-20. doi:10.1016/j. paid.2010.05.018.

205. Lindman, Ralf E., Betina M. Koskelainen, and C. J. Peter Eriksson. "Drinking, Menstrual Cycle, and Female Sexuality." *Alcoholism: Clinical & Experimental Research* 23, no. 1 (1999): 169. doi:10.1097/00000374-199901000-00025.

206. Pinker, Susan. *The Village Effect: How Face-to-face Contact Can Make Us Healthier and Happier.* Toronto: Vintage Canada, 2015.

Chapter 11

207. Bloom, Paul. *How Pleasure Works: The New Science of Why We like What We like.* New York: W.W. Norton, 2011.

208. Barash, David P. *Out of Eden the Surprising Consequences of Polygamy.* New York: Oxford University Press, 2016.

209. Bloom, Paul. *How Pleasure Works: The New Science of Why We like What We like.* New York, W.W. Norton, 2011.

210. Pincott, J. *Do Gentlemen Really Prefer Blondes?: Why He Fancies You and Why He Doesn't.* London: Bantam Press, 2008.

211. Buss, David M. *The Evolution of Desire: Strategies of Human Mating.* New York: Basic Books, 2016.

212. Bloom, Paul. *How Pleasure Works: The New Science of Why We like What We like.* New York, W.W. Norton, 2011.

213. Ibid.

214. Zak, Paul J. *Moral Molecule: How Trust Works.* NY, NY: Penguin Group, 2013.

215. Geary David. *Male, Female: The Evolution of Human Sex Differences.* Washington, D.C.: American Psychological Association, 2010.

216. Barash, David P. *Out of Eden the Surprising Consequences of Polygamy.* New York: Oxford University Press, 2016.

217. Zak, Paul J. *Moral Molecule: How Trust Works.* NY, NY: Penguin Group, 2013.

218. "Dynamic Changes in Nucleus Accumbens Dopamine Efflux During the Coolidge Effect in Male Rats" *Journal of Neuroscience*. 15 June, 1997, 17 (12) 4849-4855.

219. Zak, Paul J. *Moral Molecule: How Trust Works*. NY, NY: Penguin Group, 2013.

220. Fisher, Helen E. *Anatomy of Love: A Natural History of Mating, Marriage, and Why We Stray*. New York: W. W. Norton & Company, 2017.

Chapter 12

221. Austin Institute for Family Research, 2014.

222. Saxon, Lynn. *Sex at Dusk: Lifting the Shiny Wrapping from Sex at Dawn*. Leipzig: Amazon, 2012.

223. Hrdy, Sarah Blaffer. *Mother Nature*. New York: Pantheon, 2000.

224. Buss, David M. *The Evolution of Desire: Strategies of Human Mating*. New York: Basic Books, 2016.

225. Barash, David P. *Out of Eden the Surprising Consequences of Polygamy*. New York: Oxford University Press, 2016.

226. "Are Humans Meant to Be Monogamous?" Hopes&Fears. November 20, 2015. Accessed September 26, 2017. http://www.hopesandfears.com/hopes/now/question/216753-are-humans-meant-to-be-monogamous.

227. Ibid.

228. Lieberman, Daniel. Required to Run? Professor Proposses Harvard Bring Back Required Phys Ed. *Harvard Crimson,* August 26, 2016.

229. Buss, David M. *The Evolution of Desire: Strategies of Human Mating*. New York: Basic Books, 2016.

230. Amen, Daniel G. *Unleash the Power of the Female Brain: Supercharging Yours for Better Health, Energy,* .. Place of Publication Not Identified: Piatkus Books, 2014.

231. Hill, Napoleon. *Think and Grow Rich*. 1983, ISBN: 0449214923

232. Pinker, Susan. *The Village Effect: How Face-to-face Contact Can Make Us Healthier and Happier.* Toronto: Vintage Canada, 2015.

233. Mlodinow, Leonard. *Subliminal: How Your Unconscious Mind Rules Your Behavior*. New York: Vintage Books, 2013.

234. Ratey, John J., Richard Manning, and David Perlmutter. *Go Wild: Eat Fat, Run Free, Be Social, and Follow Evolution's Other Rules for Total Health and Well-being*. New York, NY: Little, Brown, 2015.

235. Scott, Paula Spencer. *Five Scientific Secrets for Lasting Romance*.

236. Hrdy, Sarah. *The Woman Who Never Evolved*. Cambridge: The President and Fellows of Harvard College, 1999.

237. Barash, David P. *Out of Eden the Surprising Consequences of Polygamy*. New York: Oxford University Press, 2016.

238. Fisher, Helen. Lasting Love: The Secret to Long-Term Relationships, Oprah Magazine, 2013.

239. Geher, Glenn, and Scott Barry Kaufman. *Mating Intelligence Unleashed: The Role of the Mind in Sex, Dating, and Love*. New York: Oxford University Press, 2013.

240. "The Talk: How Adults Can Promote Young People's Healthy Relationships and Prevent Misogyny and Sexual Harassment." *Making Caring Common*. Accessed November 27, 2017. https://mcc.gse.harvard.edu/thetalk.

241. Kanazawa, Satoshi. *Why More Intelligent Men (But Not Women) Value Sexual Exclusivity*. Psychology Today Online, April 19, 2010.

242. Heckman, James. "The American Family in Black and White: A Post-Racial Strategy for Improving Skills to Promote Equality." 2011. doi:10.3386/w16841.

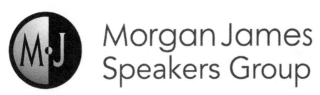

Morgan James
Speakers Group

www.TheMorganJamesSpeakersGroup.com

We connect Morgan James published authors with live and online events and audiences who will benefit from their expertise.

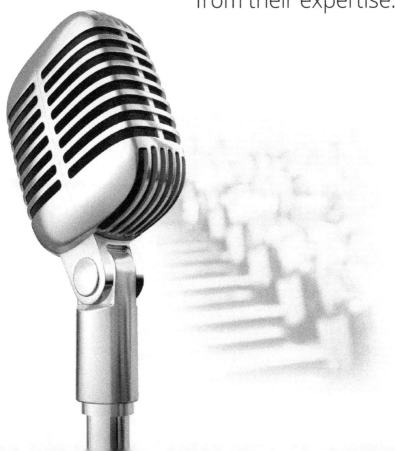

 Morgan James makes all of our titles available
through the Library for All Charity Organization.

www.LibraryForAll.org